MEDIEVAL HERBAL REM

MEDIEVAL HERBAL REMEDIES

THE *OLD ENGLISH HERBARIUM* AND ANGLO-SAXON MEDICINE

BY ANNE VAN ARSDALL

Illustrations by
Robby Poore

ROUTLEDGE
NEW YORK AND LONDON

Published in 2002 by
Routledge
270 Madison Ave,
New York NY 10016

Published in Great Britain by
Routledge
2 Park Square, Milton Park,
Abingdon, Oxon, OX14 4RN

Routledge is an imprint of the Taylor & Francis Group.

Transferred to Digital Printing 2010

Cataloging-in-Publication Data is available from the Library of Congress.

Medieval herbal remedies/Anne Van Arsdall

ISBN10: 0-415-93849-X (hbk)
ISBN10: 0-415-88403-9 (pbk)

ISBN13: 978-0-415-93849-5 (hbk)
ISBN13: 978-0-415-88403-7 (pbk)

For Aunt Mary Lou, Robby, Jonathan, and Jay

Contents

Foreword

It is a curious situation when a medieval text stands twice in need of rescue if it is to be understood and valued by modern readers, but that is the case for the *Old English Herbarium*. This medical and botanical treatise, written in the language of the Anglo-Saxons at the end of the first millennium, requires an accurate and lucid translation if it is to be used by those who value knowledge of the science and healing arts in an earlier era. Happily, Anne Van Arsdall has produced for this volume such a skilled and readable translation, based on the 1984 De Vriend edition.

Van Arsdall has, however, provided us with more than a useful translation from the Old English. She also has made clear why the *Herbarium* has been for more than a century neglected at best and misunderstood at worst, for the work has been available to those lacking specialized expertise in Old English only through the strange but influential 1864 translation and commentary by the Rev. T. Oswald Cockayne. Van Arsdall has rescued this text not only from the barriers presented to modern readers by Old English but also from the obfuscations and confusions of Cockayne's translation in his *Leechdoms, Wortcunning, and Starcraft of Early England*, the only modern English version available until the twenty-first century. In the process she has brought to light striking information about the sad life and death of this Victorian London schoolmaster. Cockayne's story calls to mind the sufferings of Dickens' fictional world as well as the intellectual milieu depicted in K. M. Elisabeth Murray's *Caught in the Web of Words* and Simon Winchester's *The Professor and the Madman*.

Although Van Arsdall's careful and vigorous translation of the Old English *Herbarium* and the strange story of Cockayne are reasons enough to value this book, her study makes other significant contributions. She sets this Anglo-Saxon work in an early-medieval medical context, and she clarifies its uses with recourse to contemporary practice of herbal medicine in Hispanic America that derives from medieval Europe.

The *Herbarium*, attributed wrongly to Apuleius Platonicus, was one of a number of Old English texts—occupying some thousand manuscript pages—that mark the first flowering of vernacular medical writing in medieval Europe. It is an expanded version of a late Roman treatise that survives in Old English in four manuscripts, one of them strikingly illustrated (British Library Cotton MSS, Vitellius C. iii). This text is by no means a mindless translation of Mediterranean herbal remedies; rather it displays practical knowledge of plants widely available in Anglo-Saxon England through cultivation and import. Van Arsdall adds to our understanding of the uses of this text by drawing on present-day *curandera* practices in the southwestern United States. She makes a cogent argument that texts like the Old English *Herbarium* served as aide-mémoire for the apprenticeship system that trains traditional healers.

This volume provides insight into the origin and uses of this remedy book of some 185 plants. It also explains its vexed reception since Cockayne's mid-nineteenth century translation, situates the *Old English Herbarium* in the context of living traditions of healing, and allows the reader to encounter it directly in a clear and graceful translation.

LINDA EHRSAM VOIGTS

Acknowledgments

My heartfelt thanks go to Professor Michael MacMahon of the University of Glasgow for his unselfish assistance in helping to obtain often hard-to-find information about Oswald Cockayne, for sharing his knowledge about the nineteenth century, and for his continued encouragement with my work. I thank Professor Maria Amalia D'Aronco of the University of Udine for supplying me with vital materials related to the *Old English Herbarium* and for sharing with me her knowledge of medieval herbals and philology. It was generous of Prof. D'Aronco to send me unpublished material to use and to help me from afar. I am indebted to Professor Linda Ehrsam Voigts of the University of Missouri at Kansas City for her guidance and encouragement as this work progressed. I am grateful to Stephanie Ball, M.D., for her willingness to answer questions about medical conditions and medical practices as well as for her enthusiasm about medieval medicine.

I thank the professors at the University of New Mexico who helped shape this study: in particular Drs. Helen Damico and Donald Sullivan, and Drs. David Bennahum, Patrick Gallacher, Claire Waters, and Gail Houston. Hats off to the staff of Interlibrary Loan at Zimmerman Library, University of New Mexico for performing miracles. I am indebted to the College of Arts and Sciences of the university for its award of an academic fellowship supporting my study. My thanks to the staff at Harvard's Houghton and Widener libraries for their helpfulness in the fall of 1998 while I was using the Cockayne collection. I am grateful to Professor Peter Bierbaumer of the University of Gratz for giving me copies of his out-of-print works on Anglo-Saxon botanical terms. At Sandia National Laboratories, for their continued support, I thank Drs. Nancy Jackson and James E. Miller, as well as my supervisors and colleagues there who often accommodated an erratic work schedule so that I could complete this work.

To my wonderful family, thank you all, not only for your support and love through it all, but for the humor that keeps me from taking myself too seriously. Special acknowledgment to my brothers Clyde and Bob, my sisters-in-law Sybil and Inez, and to my extraordinary daughters-in-law Lynne and Stacy for their never flagging encouragement, and to Isabelle and those to come, who give us hope for the future. Last but not least in the family, Mephisto, thank you for your long years of comfort. Finally, to Dr. Werner Paul Friederich, of the University of North Carolina at Chapel Hill, and to Johann Wolfgang von Goethe, my appreciation for a lifetime of inspiration.

Introduction

The *Old English Herbarium*, an Anglo-Saxon medical text from about A.D. 1000, is a translation of a fifth-century Latin work containing information on medicinal plants, the names of conditions for which they are beneficial, and directions for making remedies with them. The *Old English Herbarium* and its Latin predecessor are somewhat terse written legacies from the early-medieval period, when healing was based largely on plants and other natural substances. The work is valuable for the history of medicine because it is strikingly similar in manner of presentation, content, and seeming imprecision to modern texts on herbal medicine, a field to which modern pharmaceutical research is now turning for new or alternative therapies. A thesis advanced here is that these medical texts, medieval and modern, assume the user already has a great deal of familiarity with such material and knows how to diagnose conditions and make the remedies listed. The texts are not intended to be instructional, but are like cookbooks for experienced cooks.

For many decades, the *Herbarium* has been depicted as having been nearly useless in Anglo-Saxon England because it is a translation of a Latin work, the issue being whether the plants mentioned would have been available in the British Isles and whether the Anglo-Saxons actually used (or were capable of using) remedies from a supposedly foreign, Continental tradition. Such a depiction is demonstrated here to be erroneous, and the intent of this work is to present the *Herbarium* in a new and more positive context within the mainstream of Anglo-Saxon and European medieval healing practice. This work is structured in two parts. Part 1, comprising chapters 1 and 2, shows how a once vital medical text was transformed into a literary curiosity. Part 2, chapters 3, 4, and 5, places the *Herbarium* in an early medieval, pan-European cultural and textual tradition and interprets its contents using living traditions of herbology and modern biochemical investigations; a new translation of the *Herbarium* makes up chapter 5.

The argument presented here is that when the Rev. T. Oswald Cockayne's 1864 Rolls Series edition and translation of the *Old English Herbarium* appeared in his *Leechdoms, Wortcunning, and Starcraft of Early England*, it constituted a major transformation of what had been a book for healers. Put into a style that was controversial and antiquated even in 1864, and prefaced by biased remarks about the healing tradition to which it belonged, the *Old English Herbarium* emerged as a work that was of interest only to literary specialists. The original Latin text had been a standard reference work throughout medieval Europe, including Anglo-Saxon England, yet the preface Cockayne wrote for the Old English version of it suggests it had been of little use to the Anglo-Saxons because it was a translation from Latin and belonged to a classical or rational tradition that was alien to Anglo-Saxon healers. In addition, Cockayne's emphasis on the magical, superstitious, and other nonrational elements in the *Herbarium* and other medieval medical works has contributed to a generally negative and close-minded perception of medieval medicine generally. As discussed here, the bulk of medieval material is not superstitious or magical, but straightforward treatment using medicinal plants.

Chapter 1 presents much new material about Cockayne (1807–73), the editor and translator of the Old English medical texts, a man who experienced many disappointments in mid-nineteenth-century London. He aspired to be recognized as an Anglo-Saxon scholar and philologist, and he was a prolific writer and translator, all the while teaching classics to schoolboys in the basement rooms of King's College School. Dismissed summarily from his position when he was at an age to retire, his life ended tragically not long thereafter on the cliffs of Cornwall. His historical and cultural biases are reflected in his many works, most of which have long been forgotten but are reviewed here, together with a lost battle Cockayne fought with the eminent Joseph Bosworth, the first professor of Anglo-Saxon at Oxford. The details of Cockayne's final days, generally not known, also are here.

Chapter 2 discusses how Cockayne transformed the *Old English Herbarium* into a literary curiosity, thereby making it into what might be termed "Cockayne's *Herbarium*." The state of medicine in mid-nineteenth-century England is reviewed to depict the world of medicine during Cockayne's life; it was a state much closer to the medieval world than our own. In addition, his style of translation is shown to be attuned to the practices of the archaizing writers of his time, William Morris and Dante Gabriel Rossetti, for example, but because the style rings today (and to his time) awkwardly, arcanely, and obscurely, it makes what had been a serious medical text sound ridiculous. Finally, the chapter shows how subsequent scholars have tended wrongly to pursue and to emphasize Cockayne's suggestion that the *Old English Herbarium* was part of a classical tradition and beyond the intellectual grasp of the Anglo-Saxons, considering two other Old English works,

Bald's Leechbook and the *Lacnunga,* to be more representative of Anglo-Saxon medicine.

Chapter 3 places the Latin *Herbarium of Pseudo-Apuleius,* the original for the Old English work, into a unique medieval medical tradition, with elements drawn from classical and other sources. The *Herbarium of Pseudo-Apuleius* is a compilation that was used throughout medieval Europe, and chapter 3 shows that the medicinal plants for which it calls were available from southern Europe into the British Isles. It also draws analogies to the modern *curandera* tradition in the southwestern United States (with its roots in medieval Spain) and to modern herbology to demonstrate that the manner of healing outlined in the *Herbarium* is adaptable enough to be tailored to plants in different climates and to peoples in very different times. This tradition relies on apprenticeship with an experienced healer, knowledge of medicinal plants and how to administer them, and to a lesser extent, texts that record the plants and their use for certain conditions. For this reason, the *Herbarium* can best be understood not only from what is found in the written text, but in the context of this healing tradition, which exists today much as it did then. Finally, modern scientific approaches to the contents of the *Herbarium of Pseudo-Apuleius* and its Old English translation are showing that some of the cures are beneficial, and that in fact the uses for some of the medicinal plants may suggest new cures for the present.

Chapter 4 discusses the manuscripts in which the *Old English Herbarium* is found as well as the debates concerning its dating and possible predecessors. Discussions concerning the illustrations in MS Cotton Vitellius C iii also are reviewed briefly in this chapter. The chapter closes with an assessment of Cockayne's 1864 translation and a justification for this new one. Anyone reading Cockayne knows that a new translation is very much needed to make this text comprehensible to those who read neither Old English nor Latin and are not familiar with anachronistic nineteenth-century English. The translation relies upon experience with the modern practice of herbal medicine, drawing upon this still vital tradition to interpret the *Herbarium*'s terse directions. The underlying premise of the translator is that this is an important work, exemplifying a dynamic type of medieval medical text used throughout Europe, one that merits serious attention. Chapter 5 is a new translation of the *Old English Herbarium*, including its contents list.

The title of the work implies that the *Old English Herbarium* is an herbal (a book of plants), but instead it is a remedy book based on 185 medicinal plants, which are listed by name. Following the name are conditions the plant helps alleviate, then directions on how to administer it, either alone or with other ingredients. The classical herbal certainly is its basis, but both the *Old English Herbarium* and the Latin work from which it was translated represent another, albeit slightly different in genre, as discussed in chapter 3. In

"Herbals: Their History and Significance," George H. M. Lawrence explains the term "herbarium" as follows:

> The noun *herb* arose in the Middle Ages from the Latin *herbarius*, which was then analogous to the congener *bestarius*, the latter being a work about beasts, or animals. At that time the masculine form *herbarius* was used to identify a herb-gatherer, or herbalist, while the neuter form *herbarius* [*sic*, the editor made a mistake, the word here should be *herbarium*] was used for the place where the herbs were grown, *i.e.*, the herb garden. The herbarium of that time and well into the sixteenth century had a second definition—a place where the herbs were depicted, such as an album of drawings or illustrations of them; notes about them often would be included. A herbarium, then, could be either an herb garden or a portfolio or book. (Lawrence 1965, 3–4)

He says in later years "herbarium" was restricted to denote only a volume or portfolio of pressed or preserved plants—the antecedent of the term herbarium as it is used today. The classic herbal was more a botanical work, often illustrated, Dioscorides' *Materia Medica* and the herbals of the Renaissance being characteristic.

Seminal articles on herbals (and medieval medicine) can be found in Jerry Stannard, *Herbs and Herbalism in the Middle Ages and Renaissance* (1999a) and *Pristina Medicamenta: Ancient and Medieval Medical Botany* (1999b). Interesting general books on herbals include Agnes Arber, *Herbals: Their Origin and Evolution, A Chapter in the History of Botany, 1470–1670* (1938) and *The Illustrated Herbal* by Wilfrid Blunt and Sandra Raphael (1979).

About the Illustrations

Through the many centuries of the late classical and medieval periods, it was traditional for manuscript illustrators to base their renditions of plant, animal, and other figures on earlier works. We continue this ancient tradition here. With the facsimile edition of the *Old English Herbarium* by D'Aronco and Cameron on a drafting table beside him, artist Robby Poore (a graphic designer for the University of North Carolina at Chapel Hill) took up the challenge of making original drawings of thirty of the plants from the *Herbarium* and a representative snake and scorpion to accompany this translation. We hope the anonymous illustrators of yore will smile on our work.

1

Oswald the Obscure

The Lifelong Disappointments of T. O. Cockayne

> Where art thou, O nameless one?
> And dost thou laugh to look upon
> My eagerness thy tale to read
> Midst such changed hope and fear and need?
> Or somewhere near me dost thou stand,
> And through the dark reach out thine hand?
> Yea, are we friends?
>
> —William Morris,
> *Envoi to the Eyrbyggja Saga, 1870*

In a listing of Anglo-Saxon scholars by importance, somewhere toward the end, but certainly present, would be the Rev. T. Oswald Cockayne (1807–73). Cockayne was the first (and so far the only) person to transcribe from the original eleventh-century manuscripts and translate into modern English the three major Anglo-Saxon medical manuscripts—the *Old English Herbarium*, *Bald's Leechbook*, and the *Lacnunga*, which he published in three volumes in 1864 under the title *Leechdoms, Wortcunning, and Starcraft of Early England*.[1] This is now virtually the only work for which he is known.

Only the briefest biographical details are generally given about Cockayne's life. The following pages have the first comprehensive account to date, containing details that are not widely known, such as his enigmatic relationship with some of the British circle of more famous mid-nineteenth-century early English scholars, Henry Sweet (1845–1912), W. W. Skeat (1835–1912), and Joseph Bosworth (1789–1876). Also of interest is that by 1878, only a few years after Cockayne's death, the American book collector William Medlicott already owned most of Cockayne's personal library and some of his handwritten notebooks. When Medlicott offered his extensive library for sale that year, Harvard purchased most of the Cockayne material, and it remains in the Houghton and Widener Libraries.[2]

The facts of Cockayne's life are the stuff of a bittersweet Victorian novel. An ordained minister, Cockayne obtained a master's degree in 1835 when he was twenty-eight, and seven years later he became a schoolmaster, teaching Latin, Greek, and mathematics in the basement rooms of a boy's school in London. There he stayed for twenty-seven years (1842–69), when he was summarily dismissed from his position at the age of sixty-two without a pension. Only a few years later, in 1873, he allegedly committed suicide. When mention is made of Cockayne today, he is generally assumed to have been an eminent nineteenth-century Anglo-Saxon scholar, but the details of his life do not bear out this assumption. His feat in transcribing and translating the Old English medical texts, together with his other laborious and now overlooked contributions to scholarship, become all the more monumental when the facts about his tragic life are known.

Cockayne, the Philologist: The Lost Battle with Bosworth

Before translating the *Old English Herbarium* in the early 1860s, Cockayne published an odd assortment of works: *Civil History of the Jews* (1845), *A Greek Syntax with Metrical Examples* (1846), *History of France* (1848; second revised edition 1850), *History of Ireland for Families and Schools* (1851), and *Life of Marshal Turenne* (1858). His *Civil History of the Jews,* which saw two editions in 1845, showed him to be a biblical literalist: "Sacred and profane history spring from separate fountains, and flow in separate streams, and yet they unite in certain particulars to prove that the miracles of the Exodus are real events."[3] Cockayne's expressed intent in writing the work was to locate exactly where biblical events occurred, quoting from such sources as, for example, "Mr. Burckhardt's Travels in Syria of 1822" and "Ignatius of Rheinfelden" from 1656 to shed light on biblical stories using the type of citations popular in the nineteenth century: cryptic author names of mostly forgotten works at the bottom of the page, sometimes with a volume or page number, often without, for example, "Mr. Clinton's Fasti, vol. 1." Though he did not say it in so many words, Cockayne obviously thought little had changed in the Holy Land since the time of the prophets.

Cockayne's scholarly interests, mirrored in his publications, turned to Anglo-Saxon studies with a passion—the early 1860s marked a flurry of works on philology and Old English. He published two philological works, *Spoon and Sparrow* (1861) and *Narratiunculae Anglice Conscriptae* (1861),[4] and three translations/editions for the Early English Text Society, *Ste. Marherete the Meiden ant Martyr* (1862), *Hali Meidenhad* (1866), and *Juliana* (1872) with Edmund Brock. The three-volume *Leechdoms, Wortcunning, and Starcraft of Early England,* published in the Rolls Series (1864–66) later became Cockayne's best known work. Appearing intermittently was *The Shrine: A Collection of Papers on Dry Subjects, in 13 Parts* (1864–70),[5] presenting short essays and transcriptions of Old English texts. The quaintness of his original titles mirrored his penchant for an arcane style of translation and a love of older languages.

Cockayne's publications on philology give an insight into the field of Early English studies as it was developing in the mid-to-late-1800s and reveal a particular *Weltanschauung* from the middle of the Victorian Age, rooted in a literal interpretation of the Bible, just as the Darwinian theory of evolution—and concurrently theories of language evolution—were emerging. This was a seminal era for linguistics, the connection between Sanskrit and the European languages having been asserted, challenged, and generally accepted. Considerable discussion then ensued in terms of explaining the connection between languages, when the possible relationship of Western languages to Sanskrit and Hebrew was being debated—but Cockayne was not in the mainstream of the debate.[6] The important element for him was that any linguistic study had to be compatible with a literal interpretation of the Bible, and his real interest in languages was cultural, not linguistic. He preferred to focus on social customs and the evolution of meaning as found in written texts, not on descriptions of language change and language families apart from the texts.

Spoon and Sparrow[7] was Cockayne's major, if unheralded, contribution to linguistics and philology. He stated in it that an early form of Teutonic coexisted with Homeric Greek, Phoenician, biblical Hebrew, Latin, and Sanskrit. He reasoned that because the world's languages were differentiated by the Lord at Babel, the changes in language groups could be traced to this event. For him, a key to understanding these changes was word borrowing, and vocabulary is the important word here. Cockayne's quest was to establish word families and to trace who borrowed what word from whom. He soundly rejected derivational explanations: "Nobody, it may be presumed, is bound to pin his faith upon all that everybody has said about derivations from the sanskrit. . . . Latin and greek words must be like the sanskrit both in shape and sense, and variations must in some way explained or paralleled, or else the comparison is unconvincing" (*Spoon*, 4).[8]

Rather than seeking to formulate general laws, Cockayne used a plethora of invented rules to distinguish borrowed words from what he called "true parallels." In his publications, Cockayne was very much the Victorian scholar in using no footnotes, no explanation of the reasons behind his pronouncements, and no appeal to any authority but his own judgment. His study of words resembles somewhat the method for compiling the *Oxford English Dictionary* and its quest to ascertain the original meaning of words in English (and Cockayne liked to point out wrong usage).

Cockayne's etymological method, if it can be called that, is not easy to follow; a typical explanation is the following:

Some instinctive tests exist by which to discriminate between borrowed words and true parallels. Thus compounds can hardly be accepted [as true parallels?] . . . Afformative letters added to the visible root afford a strong ground of suspicion. Yet I would say "instinctive tests" rather than rules, for it is not reasonable to suppose but that old roots had acquired some afformative letters while still some of the kindred nations were undivided from each other. (*Spoon*, 7)

One or two principles may seem here sometimes to be tacitly assumed without proof; one is, that in the same syllables, or more exactly, in varied forms of equivalents, that which retains the greater number of letters is the more ancient. . . . [I]n such instances as May, Μεγαλα (pl.), Magnus, the shorter form of May [i.e., the English word] is older, having none of the afformative syllables of the others. In this instance a root which to Homer 800 B.C. had perished, and was dead of age, still survives in the common talk of England. (*Spoon*, 8)

Cockayne's personal sense of the original languages, Teutonic among them, was his major justification for conclusions about what must have been the original words in Teutonic and other languages. His supposed proofs of relationships among words across language families are actually descriptions of how words might be assumed to be related based on comparisons of vaguely similar meaning. *Spoon and Sparrow* has nearly a thousand numbered paragraphs, each illustrating findings such as those provided in the examples above.

Cockayne did not know that he was considering words in languages from quite different ages and at various developmental stages, a factor the newer German-based linguistics was beginning to recognize. The concept was emerging of a parent language (Indo-European) behind even Sanskrit and ancient Greek for a certain number of the world's languages, not for all of them, and the new concepts did not involve a need for Babel. Indeed, it was becoming extremely difficult by 1861, when *Spoon and Sparrow* was published, to reconcile common reckonings of time based on the Bible and what linguistics was demonstrating. This was a period when the traditional world view based on the biblical account was under siege on all fronts and was slowly giving way to a new one based on Darwin and evolution. Cockayne was not alone in clinging to the old.

Cockayne maintained that (at least when he was living) much of English usage had, in fact, never been written down, and to back himself up, cited several words and phrases used in the countryside that were not in any dictionary. For this reason, he thought many ancient Teutonic words also remained unknown. Here may be the major reason Cockayne chose to transcribe and translate the Anglo-Saxon medical texts; he may have hoped to find a medical or plant vocabulary that was unique to Teutonic. At paragraph twenty-three in *Spoon and Sparrow*, he makes the interesting observation:

The deficiencies of the vocabulary of anglosaxon books are supplied by glossaries. How many must have been the words that Ælfric never heard, how many that he refused to admit when he did hear them, how many that did not present themselves while compiling a glossary. A small examination of unpublished manuscripts will soon convince any one who can read the language, that the admirable industry of Lye and Manning had not completed the whole task: nor has any one equal to the undertaking yet appeared. . . . Modern lexicon makers are not to be named in the same page as the old heroes of this battle. (*Spoon*, 10)

Edward Lye (1694–1767) did not live to see the publication of his *Dictionarium saxonico et gothico-latinum*, which was edited and published with his memoirs in 1772 by Owing Manning (1721–1801). One biographer in the *British Biographical Archives* called Lye "a learned divine," and his dictionary was a standard authority in the nineteenth century. Cockayne, W. W. Skeat, and others always referred to it simply as Lye and Manning. The modern "lexicon maker" to whom Cockayne refers here is Prof. Joseph Bosworth, whose *Anglo-Saxon Dictionary* appeared in 1838.

Nearly buried toward the end of *Spoon and Sparrow* is a statement by the author that reveals the keen disappointment Cockayne must have felt most of his life, after sifting through uncounted numbers of words in so many languages, producing so many works, teaching, and being virtually ignored. He was clearly thwarted in his desire to be recognized as a philologist. He wrote here that he wanted to gain the reader's confidence by testing his own theories on numerals and some common proper names. "That I am surprised at the results would be a small thing to say; though they are imperfect and partial, *I trust that they will win the assent of all scholars in Europe: and if so, they cannot fail to lead on to an application of the ordinary principles of philology* in the case of the hebrew, and to bring it more or less within the reach of illustration from other tongues" [emphasis added] (*Spoon*, 265). *Spoon and Sparrow* certainly did not garner Cockayne the assent of many— if any—scholars in Europe, and its author continued to be largely ignored.

Cockayne may have modeled *Spoon and Sparrow* on Professor Joseph Bosworth's 1836 *The Origin of the Germanic and Scandinavian Languages*, which was also organized into numbered paragraphs. Bosworth was a well-known authority on Anglo-Saxon at the time, being the first professor of the subject at Oxford and the editor of a dictionary of Old English, a publication over which he and Cockayne would soon spar, as discussed below. There is no doubt that Cockayne knew Bosworth's publications. In *The Origin of the Germanic Languages*, Bosworth showed himself to be a biblical literalist like Cockayne and many people of his day, at one point stating: "The minute investigation of language is not only important in examining the mental powers, but in bearing its testimony to the truth of Revelation, and in tracing the origin and affinity of nations."[9] Bosworth explained that at Babel, the Lord confused the *pronunciation* of an original language so that people could not understand one another. His explanation of language change was more suited to the linguistic reasoning of the German school than Cockayne's, even if in particulars Bosworth was not entirely correct. Consequently, Bosworth was able to accept the new linguistics much more readily than Cockayne.

The year that *Spoon and Sparrow* was published, Cockayne suffered a major disappointment. He applied for an honorary title from King's College and was turned down. Yet by the time he petitioned for the honorary title, Cockayne had published *Narratiunculae Anglice Conscriptae* and *Spoon and Sparrow*, both of them philological works, and he was at work on an edition/translation of the Old English *Seinte Marherete*. The procedure for granting an honorary title had recently been created at the University College of London at the time Cockayne made his request, so the request would not have been unusual.[10] Among the few details Charles Singer offers about Cockayne is the college's refusal to grant him ". . . the title of Honorary Professor of Philology in the College, though he had well earned it by his writings" (Singer in Cockayne 1961, 1:xvii). About the same time (1861–62), records of the Philological Society show that Cockayne left the society, which he had joined in 1843, a year after its foundation. His resignation is surprising, because this society was at the center of the linguistic/philological debate, and its members encompassed the leading philologists in England. What may have happened to cause him to leave the society and whether the reason or reasons were connected with the denial of his honorary title is not clear, but the two events were so close in time, they almost certainly were related and did not bode well for his fortunes as a scholar of early English.

In spite of these personal setbacks, Cockayne began to transcribe and translate the major Anglo-Saxon medical manuscripts, which the Rolls Series published as *Leechdoms, Wortcraft, and Starcunning of Early England* in three volumes from 1864–66. It is unfortunate that the publication records of the *Leechdoms*, part of the Longman's Company archives housed at Reading University, have disappeared, apparently destroyed during bombings in World War II. G. Michael C. Bott of the Reading library related: "It is curious not to find a ledger entry [on Cockayne's volumes] since the series of ledgers, commission and divide, are unbroken (despite the fires!) from ca. 1800; curious too that Cockayne's volumes are not mentioned in Longman's trade magazine *Notes on Books* which starts in the 1850s."[11] It would be interesting to know whether the Rolls Series approached Cockayne to do the work or whether he offered to do it, and whether he was paid.

Evidence from Cockayne's personal notebooks at Harvard and essays published in *The Shrine* show him to have been extremely interested in the vocabulary of the Anglo-Saxons. In fact he clearly believed he was a more reliable authority on the vocabulary and language of Old English than

Bosworth, because at about this time, 1863–64, he tried unsuccessfully to become part of the Anglo-Saxon dictionary that Bosworth was revising.

It seems that Cockayne sent a letter to Oxford University demanding he be named joint or chief editor of the dictionary with his name on its title page, saying he expected to be well paid for his services. If Oxford did not meet his demands, Cockayne said he would publish a pamphlet about Bosworth's deficient knowledge of Old English. He even sent Bosworth a draft of the text, saying he planned to send it further "to all the Reviews and to men of influence in Oxford and London," a quote from a defense of Bosworth that was published soon after Cockayne made good on his threat and published the anti-Bosworth pamphlet.[12] It appears that Cockayne never received a reply to his demands from anyone, and in 1864, he published "Dr. Bosworth and His Saxon Dictionary" in *The Shrine*. Cockayne subsequently never denied having made the demands.

C. B. Thurston, an Oxford associate of Bosworth's, explained in his nineteen-page-long *A Few Remarks in Defense of Dr. Bosworth* that no reply was sent to Cockayne because his accusations were so off-base, nobody thought Cockayne would dare publish them. Thurston gave the reason for Bosworth's silence as "the style and spirit of the [Cockayne's] whole pamphlet, which appeared a sufficient answer, especially in Oxford, where the high tone of gentlemanly feeling, which pervades the whole University, cannot endure such assumptions and personalities; he [Bosworth] therefore let the matter rest" (Thurston, 5).

Much later, J. J. R. Tolkien quoted from Cockayne's attack on Bosworth to begin his landmark 1936 lecture, "*Beowulf*: The Monsters and the Critics": "In 1864 the Reverend Oswald Cockayne wrote of the Reverend Doctor Joseph Bosworth, Rawlinsonian Professor of Anglo-Saxon: 'I have tried to lend to others the conviction I have long entertained that Dr. Bosworth is not a man so diligent in his special walk as duly to read the books . . . which have been printed in our old English, or so-called Anglosaxon tongue. He may do very well for a professor.' These words were inspired by dissatisfaction with Bosworth's dictionary, and were doubtless unfair."[13]

More than dissatisfaction, indeed, deep-seated anger appears to have prompted Cockayne to publish eleven pages of bitter indictments in "Dr. Bosworth and His Saxon Dictionary," beginning "Should it be made clear . . . that any new edition prepared by Dr. Bosworth can hardly be free from grave errors, it must be the most anxious wish of all who respect that most noble home and nursery of learning, that the responsibility for those errors shall rest with Dr. Bosworth alone [and not be associated with Oxford]" (*Shrine*, 1). While admitting that Bosworth's 1855 *Compendious Anglo-Saxon Dictionary* had some merit, Cockayne questioned what readers might expect from a new and improved edition, surmising the new edition might now to its detriment include linguistics (philology for Cockayne), saying ". . . but it is not comparative philology (filology) nor Bopp nor Pott nor an army of German fanatics in languages, that we want in a Saxon Dictionary. We look for a work that shall reassure young students, that shall shew them their way in old English sentences, that shall convince them that our old tongue was grammatical and that its periods will bear the ordinary tests" (*Shrine*, 2). The "German fanatics" to whom Cockayne refers were Franz Bopp (1791–1867) and August Friedrich Pott (1802–87). Bopp was a well-known German linguist who published his *Analytical Comparison of the Sanskrit, Greek, Latin, and Teutonic Languages* in 1816, looking particularly at the grammatical structure of these languages. He continued to add more languages to what was emerging as an Indo-European language group. The place of Sanskrit in this scheme was debated—was it the parent language or a brother to Latin and Greek? Bopp took the brother approach; some like August Schleicher sought an *Ursprache* (possibly Sanskrit) and wrote about languages in terms of youth, maturity, and decay, a theory that was mirrored by many historians of the time about the evolution of societies. Pott wrote *Einleitung in die Allgemeine Sprachwissenschaft*, but was not as well known as Bopp.

Cockayne then turned his attention in the attack to Bosworth's credentials, saying that he doubted whether the Oxford professor of Anglo-Saxon had even bothered to read any Anglo-Saxon or the standard authors on the subject:

> Up to this point I have tried to lend to others the conviction I have long entertained, that Dr. Bosworth is not a man so diligent in his special walk, as duly to read the books, especially the Gospels, which have been printed in our old English, or so called Anglosaxon, tongue. He may do very well for a Professor, but before the University of Oxford shares with him the title page of a dictionary I will try to make my voice, feeble as I know it to be, heard on the other side. Let me now proceed to prove, if I can, that in 1855 when he published his Compendious Dictionary he was unacquainted with Kembles Codex Diplomaticus published ten years before. (*Shrine*, 4)

The major allegation was Bosworth's incorrect assignments of gender to nouns, for example: "Baec, a beck, Kemble in the Codex published in 1845 marks masculine. Under the spelling in 1855 Dr. Bosworth does not seem to know it; under Becc no gender is assigned. Did he despise the scholarship of J. M. Kemble, or had he never, ten years afterwards, seen his book?" (*Shrine*, 7).

Cockayne asserted that in 1855 Bosworth was "ill acquainted with the literature of which he made a dictionary" (*Shrine*, 9) and said it was no wonder that Bosworth "who has not had time, in better than seventy years, to read our classical Old English, should be not very well up in the glossaries" (*Shrine*, 11). Cockayne challenged Bosworth to reply to each of the charges and to prove he had "done his duty as a lexicografer." The attack closed:

> Against Dr. Bosworth I have no further grudge, than what one feels towards
> a man who has not done his work well. I have just put out of hand a volume
> in which some errors he has committed, none of them here mentioned, were
> corrected without bringing his name in all. But I find myself unable to stand
> by, silent, when the name of the University of Oxford is to be put on the title
> page of such a book as he shall make. (*Shrine*, 11)

The anger and resentment in these remarks tempt speculation that Bosworth
might have been behind the refusal in granting Cockayne the honorary title in
1861 and that Cockayne might have known it.

The reply did not come from Professor Bosworth directly; in his pamphlet defending Bosworth, Thurston said the professor was "determined not
to notice it" (Thurston, 4). As Thurston elaborated on the scenario, Bosworth
was told that a Mr. Cockayne was preparing a pamphlet against the dictionary and inquired who this Mr. Cockayne was. Choosing his words carefully,
Thurston said they ascertained that Cockayne was one of the undermasters at
King's College School, London, thus clearly establishing Cockayne's lowly
status vis-á-vis the Oxford Professor. Yet by this time, Cockayne had published part of the *Leechdoms*, the *Narratiunculae Anglice Conscripitae*,
Spoon and Sparrow, and *Seinte Marherete* for the EETS, and had been an
active member of the Philological Society.

Thurston said he used Bosworth's notes to reply to each of Cockayne's
accusations, asserting that Bosworth read Anglo-Saxon manuscripts at an
early age and copied out numerous passages from manuscripts at the British
Museum and elsewhere for his first Anglo-Saxon dictionary, published in
1838. Thurston questioned the dates Cockayne assigned to Bosworth's large
dictionary, saying it was published in 1848, not 1855, stating:

> . . . it is clear that Mr. Cockayne was so little acquainted with Anglo-Saxon
> literature and bibliography in the year 1855, as not to know that this Com-
> pendious Dictionary was published in 1848. It proves . . . that his Anglo-
> Saxon studies have not been close, nor minute, nor of long duration, not
> having commenced before 1855, and perhaps some years later. His time,
> therefore, limited as it is by his scholastic duties, would leave very little
> opportunity for a careful reading of the numerous MSS in the British
> Museum, exclusive of those in Oxford and Cambridge. (Thurston, 7)

There was, however, indeed an 1855 *edition* of the Bosworth dictionary
(if admittedly not the original edition), and Harvard's Widener Library owns
Cockayne's annotated copy of it.

In the pamphlet, Thurston correctly criticized Cockayne for being "unable
to rise above the consideration of genders and conjugations" (Thurston, 9),
saying the prevailing feature of Cockayne's attack was a depreciation of others
and praise of himself. Thurston concluded the pamphlet as follows:

I have, I believe, succeeded in showing that Mr. Cockayne is—
Wrong in his dates; and therefore
Wrong in the conclusions he draws from those dates;
Wrong as to his statement of errors;
Wrong as to the knowledge of the Gospels;
Wrong as to the omission of genders;
Wrong in the genders of nouns;
Wrong in the meaning of brecan and brecende;
Wrong in the meaning of English *beholden*, and its application;
Wrong in the meaning of the Anglo-Saxon behealdan; and
Wrong in his supposed influence with the University of Oxford; and that
therefore, his judgement on a literary work is as worthless as his attempt to
interfere with an existing arrangement is unjustifiable. (Thurston, 18)

There was a sequel to this particular incident. That same year, 1864,
Cockayne replied to Thurston in *The Shrine*, volume 3, where his "Postscript
on Bosworth's Dictionary" began, "To some private representations, I reply,
that in Dr. Bosworth's dictionary I see just the small merit that I admitted; it
is no more trustworthy of footing than a Welsh bog." He called the reply
"noisy and unsubstantial" (but did not name Thurston) and offered more
from his "stock of Bosworthian blunders" (*Shrine*, 24). Not only did he continue the accusations about Bosworth, he included the German philologist
Christian Wilhelm Michael Grein (1825–77), about whom he said
". . . edited the texts without critical acuteness; and his dictionary may be
truly 'admirable' to our Oxford lexicon maker, but it is at first sight no great
thing to others" (*Shrine*, 26–7). Cockayne ended by saying that he could not
abide or tolerate in the Bosworth reply what he called "audacious volunteer-
ing, the gratuitous speculation, the unlawful enterprise" (*Shrine*, 27). The
exchange appears to have ended here, but it was clearly prompted by more
than scholarly concern on the part of Cockayne. He took on a lion of the
establishment, and, to add to his other disappointments, did not even merit a
personal reply. Instead, an underling was sent into the fray, and the battle
royal for Cockayne was merely a minor tiff for Bosworth.

Why Cockayne turned later in his life to Anglo-Saxon as the focus of his
scholarship is uncertain, because at heart he appeared to have always cher-
ished the culture and literature of the classical world and to have regarded the
world of the Germanic tribes with a certain amount of disdain. In particular,
when speaking of the early Germanic world, Cockayne frequently referred to
the Teutonic tribes coming in contact with the "superior" race and civilization of Rome and Greece. Moreover, Cockayne offered few comments on
original Anglo-Saxon poetry or prose literature other than saints' lives, even
though he owned and annotated a copy of Benjamin Thorpe's 1855 edition of
Beowulf (currently in the Harvard collection), and scattered references to
other original Old English works can be found, but none with any judgment

on their quality. On the other hand, Cockayne dealt at length with Gawin Douglas's translation of the *Aeneid* into Middle Scots.[14] His extensive remarks about the translation are found in a cardboard-bound notebook at Harvard (MS ENG 641).

It might be argued that all Cockayne's translations from Old English, including those of the three saints' lives, served pragmatic, not literary, purposes; they centered on virginity and virtue, geography, magico-medicine, and charms. In fact, at Harvard is a leather-bound, blank book belonging to Cockayne of much better quality than the cardboard-bound notebooks on file there. In it, he had carefully allotted pages to each letter of the alphabet, writing the letters in ink at the top of the page, and had begun making notes throughout the book on Anglo-Saxon geographical names, obviously with the intention of continuing the work for many years.

Cockayne acquired considerable linguistic ability in Old English, and he was continually concerned with exactness in dealing with it, witness his obvious alarm at Bosworth's continued success in publishing what he considered faulty material. It is noteworthy that Cockayne and Bosworth were both trained classicists; indeed, Bosworth published a text on translating Latin that went through several editions.[15] Whereas Cockayne remained a teacher of classics in a boys' school, Bosworth gained some fame and a doctoral degree while living in Holland (1829–40), returning to England and several vicarages, then being named Rawlinson Professor of Anglo-Saxon at Oxford in 1857, about the time Cockayne appears to have begun to be seriously engaged in studying and writing about Anglo-Saxon. Bosworth's *Anglo-Saxon Dictionary*, first published in 1838, and his other writings on Old English are reported to have earned him 18,000 pounds sterling over the years, a very large sum at the time and enough to enable him in 1867 to endow a professorship of Anglo-Saxon at Cambridge, Cockayne's alma mater. Remarks by W. W. Skeat and Henry Sweet cited later in this chapter show that Bosworth was not always praised without reservation as a scholar, and his biography by Henry Bradley in the standard *Dictionary of National Biography* is fairly critical. Bradley (1845–1925), a philologist and lexicographer, was an editor of the *Oxford English Dictionary.* Interestingly enough, Bradley's entry on Bosworth cites Cockayne's *Shrine* as one of its sources (the publication in which the attack on Bosworth had appeared).

But if Bosworth's scholarship, his ideas on etymology and linguistics, even the dictionary for which he is so famous can be correctly judged as flawed, yet he did not infuse his work with bias favoring Rome and Greece and against the Anglo-Saxon world. Bosworth's work revolved around his interest in philology and linguistics, and he did not stray far from it in his publications. In contrast to Cockayne's prefaces to the *Leechdoms*, the preface to one of Bosworth's earliest publications, *Elements of Anglo-Saxon*

Grammar (1823), revealed Bosworth's admiration for the barbarian speakers of Anglo-Saxon and established them as the founding fathers, as it were, of British civilization:

> We have insensibly imbibed the opinions of the Roman authors which we have read, and, with the name of Goths, have constantly associated every species of ignorance, cruelty, and barbarity; not considering that we, as Englishmen, are indebted to the descendants of the Gothic tribes for our existence, our language, and our laws.[16]

Bosworth's *Anglo-Saxon Dictionary* went through many printings in his lifetime and has been a standard for many years despite its drawbacks (after his death it was revised and enlarged by T. Northcote Toller and printed again in 1882).

Cockayne, on the other hand, although publishing and attempting to publish on many of the same subjects as Bosworth, saw less success. Few of his publications are read today—with the notable exception of the *Leechdoms*. Unfortunately, and unlike Bosworth's works, the *Leechdoms* was written from the vantage point of a classicist examining the rude world of the northern Germans, and it established a biased foundation for much modern writing about Anglo-Saxon medicine in particular and the medieval medical tradition generally, as explored further in subsequent chapters.

Cockayne's *Leechdoms, Wortcunning, and Starcraft of Early England*

Why then, did Cockayne undertake this massive work? He may have been seeking as-yet-undiscovered vocabulary from the Teutonic world by looking at the medical manuscripts. Or, perhaps this unveiling of what he called superstition and folly would vindicate his attitude toward the Anglo-Saxon world—possibly it helped shape that attitude; perhaps in translating these three magico-medical texts he wanted to set the record straight about the culture of these Anglo-Saxons. It is no matter of chance that volume 1 of this series on "science before the Norman conquest" opens: "It will be difficult for the kindliest temper to give a friendly welcome to the medical philosophy of Saxon days" (Cockayne 1965, 1:ix). He portrayed the Germanic tribes as being in awe of Rome, which may be true, but then stated that they were incapable of mastering much of what the superior civilization offered, extending that prejudice to the corpus of early medieval medical texts:

> Not only the Engle and Seaxe, the warrior inhabitants of our own island, but all the races of Gothic invaders, were too rude to learn much of Gallenos, or of Alexander of Tralles, though they would fain do so. The writings of Marcellus, called Empericus, the Herbarium of Apuleius, the stuff current under

the name of Sextus Placitus, the copious volumes of Constantinus Africanus, the writings of St. Hildegard of Bingen, the collections out of Dioskorides, the smaller Saxon pieces, are all of one character, substituting for the case of instruments and Indian drugs, indigenous herbs, the worts of the fatherland, smearings, and wizard chants. Over the whole face of Europe . . . the next to hand remedy became the established remedy, and the searching incision of the practiced anatomist was replaced by a droning song. (Cockayne 1965, 1:xxvii)

The following chapter includes a discussion of how Cockayne transformed what had been a respected and much used early medieval medical text into a literary curiosity. It shows how the *Herbarium of Pseudo-Apuleius* (in its Anglo-Saxon version known as the *Old English Herbarium*) and the other Anglo-Saxon medical texts became in his hands objects of ridicule and examples of superstition. Not only the transformation of medical texts into curiosities, but the world of misconceptions about medieval medical practices suggested by Cockayne would be taken over and greatly amplified by Charles Singer, as discussed in chapter 2. Cockayne's training, profession, and most of all, his personal preferences in culture and literature help explain the attitude with which he approached all the Anglo-Saxon medical texts and, despite his linguistic exactitude, reveal him to have been prejudiced toward the culture that spoke Anglo-Saxon (whereas Bosworth apparently was not, though both men shared similar backgrounds and scope of interests).

Cockayne's merit as an Anglo-Saxonist was questioned by the Bosworth exchange, his philological works went unnoticed, and so too did his translations, even the *Leechdoms, Wortcunning, and Starcraft of Early England* for which he is known today. The *Leechdoms* represent enormous effort. They are primarily philological works on Anglo-Saxon culture, whose purpose is revealed in the prefaces Cockayne wrote to each of its three volumes, where as mentioned, he discussed the early Germanic peoples from the vantage point of a clearly superior civilization, looking rather fondly at the English people in their childhood days.

The longest preface he wrote was for volume 1, which contains his transcription and translation of the *Old English Herbarium*. The 105 pages of his preface cover Greek, Roman, and early Germanic and Anglo-Saxon medicine, and they generally lambast early Germanic medical lore and practices and praise the classical. Among other notions that Cockayne introduced here is the idea that superstitious practices, such as incantations and amulets, although not absent in classical times, became more prevalent as the Germanic nations overcame the Roman Empire. He devoted a number of pages to examples of what he clearly considered ridiculous treatments for various ailments throughout the Middle Ages, contrasting them at many points with the classical approach and lamenting the loss of medical and surgical knowledge from the ancients. He even suggested that Anglo-Saxon healers did not believe in what they wrote: "Possibly the makers of magic gibberish [the Saxon leeches] were as incredulous as men are now in its efficacy: but what mattered that? The leechbook must adapt itself to its day" (Cockayne 1965, 1:xxxiii). This preface shares the muddled organization, lack of coherence, and pompous style of *Spoon and Sparrow*.

Volume 2 of the *Leechdoms* contains the three books that make up *Bald's Leechbook*, another medical text that is roughly contemporary with the *Old English Herbarium*. Cockayne's preface says very little about the *Leechbook*, and instead discusses what he termed the manners and customs of the Anglo-Saxons, defending the Saxons against charges that they were "mangy dogs. . . . [R]oving savages [who] stuffed their bellies with acorns" (Cockayne 1965, 2:vii). In fact, he painted quite a detailed and favorable picture of the early Saxons and their food, medicines, and drink, saying that he was here drawing together in one place "scattered notices" about this subject. The footnotes are characteristically vague and hard to connect to actual works, all of them primary sources, but it is also very clear that Cockayne did *not* mention Sharon Turner's *The History of the Anglo-Saxons* (1799–1805), which he certainly knew and occasionally cited by name in his other writings.[17] Turner's volume 3 covers "The Manners of the Anglo-Saxons after Their Occupation of England" and it contains information on food, medicine, customs, and education, the same topics Cockayne treated later. Though he quibbled with Turner about details of the Anglo-Saxon language, he clearly shared Turner's concept of history, a concept that is fundamental to understanding *Spoon and Sparrow* and especially Cockayne's prefaces and notes to the *Leechdoms*.

This concept views all known history as being subsequent to the Flood, which happened at about 2348 B.C. At that time, the human race was renewed, and very early, these people (who were in a state of civilized perfection) began to separate into the civilized and nomadic nations; in Turner's words: ". . . from hence [the nomadic peoples] first spread into those wilder and ruder districts, where nature was living in all her unmolested, but dreary, and barbarous majesty."[18] It was natural that the nomadic peoples change as they migrated, and some (notably the Celts) sank into absolute barbarism. Others, like the Teutonic tribes, though living a rough and vigorous life, managed to maintain the highest moral code and the best of what they took with them from civilization.

While the nomadic migrations were underway, many of the civilized nations, as Turner put it "degenerated into sensuality, into debasing vices, and to effeminate frivolities" (Turner, 1:11). Turner devoted three volumes to the establishment of the Anglo-Saxons in England, seeing the result this way:

> But the Saxons were one of those obscure tribes whom Providence was training up to establish more just governments, more improving institu-

tions, and more virtuous, though fierce manners, in the corrupted and incorrigible population of imperial Rome. And they advanced from their remote, almost unknown corridor of ancient Germany, with a steady and unreceding progress, to the distinguished destiny to which they were conducted. (Turner, 1:116)

Echoes of Turner are found throughout Cockayne's writings, though Cockayne expressed much greater preference than Turner for Roman and Greek accomplishments in comparison with the Anglo-Saxon world.

Another source Cockayne failed to list by author and title is Thomas Wright's *A Volume of Vocabularies, Illustrating the Condition and Manners of Our Forefathers as Well as the History of the Forms of Elementary Education and of the Languages Spoken in this Island, from the Tenth Century to the Fifteenth* (1857). Cockayne's personal copy of this book is at Harvard's Houghton Library; it is a copy with the signature of O. Cockayne on the inside front cover, in pencil, with the date 1863. Wright's book contains many of the texts that Cockayne said he used for this preface (and for the other prefaces). If Cockayne was guilty of omitting at least these two sources, he was certainly not guilty of neglecting to cite his own works; he listed the *Leechdoms*, *Spoon and Sparrow*, *The Shrine*, and *Narratiunculae* as sources used in writing the prefaces.

Cockayne summarized *Bald's Leechbook* in this way:

> Notwithstanding that this is a learned book, it sometimes sinks to mere driveling. The author almost always rejects the Greek recipes, and doctors as an herborist. It will give any one who has the heart of a man in him a thrill of horror to compare the Saxon dose of brooklime and pennyroyal twice a day, for a mother whose child is dead within her, with the chapter in Celsus devoted to this subject, in which we read, as in his inmost soul, an anxious courageous care, and a sense of responsibility mixed with determination to do his utmost . . . (Cockayne 1965, 2:xx)

It would be vain to defend these prescriptions, Cockayne asserted, saying that Saxon leeches tried to qualify themselves for their profession by searching the medical records of classical cultures.

Volume 3 of the *Leechdoms* contains *Lacnunga*, an Anglo-Saxon book on medicinal plants and healing remedies with many chants and incantations. In addition are smaller works, the ΠΕΡΙ ΔΙΔΑΞΕΩΝ (About Schools), "On the Formation of the Foetus," a section titled "Starcraft" containing "prognostics from the moon's age, a [Sun] "Dial," "On the Calendar," a "Treatise on Astronomy and Cosmogony" by Bede; a section on charms; and a curious addition with a long preface containing miscellaneous historical pieces. Also in this volume is a glossary of Saxon names of plants, as well as the "Durham Glossary of the Names of Worts." In the preface to this particular volume, a haughty Cockayne wrote: "in the collection now printed we are allowed an insight into the notions and prepossessions upon scientific subjects of the less instructed portion of Saxon society. The unfounded hopes, scruples, and alarms of the ignorant, ignorant by comparison [with the Saxons who sought classical learning], are justly regarded by the wise with a copious contempt" (Cockayne 1965, 3:vii–viii). An overview of heathen Saxon mythology, a lengthy, rambling discourse on dream lore, and finally a history of astrology and healing with a long passage about the books of Hermes make up most of the preface. More than ten pages are then devoted to Ælfric's writings and a discussion of who Ælfric might have been. It is not clear how or whether the discussion relates to the texts in this volume, other than an opening remark that "the authorship of the translation or adaptation of the work of Bede de Temporibus has been attributed to the grammarian Ælfric."(Cockayne 1965, 3:xiv). Volume 3 contains the Anglo-Saxon version of Bede's *De Temporibus*, but it is a small portion of the works collected there.

Singer may have been correct about Cockayne's prefaces being out of date, his reason for dropping them and substituting his own in his 1961 reprint of the *Leechdoms*. However, without them, the true flavor and intent of the translator is lost. The three prefaces show Cockayne not as a student of Anglo-Saxon or medieval medicine, nor as a seeker of knowledge about plants and how they might have been used since Greek times, nor as an impartial translator of practical medical treatises, but more as a member of a clearly superior civilization looking into the follies of long ago. Whatever purpose he had in doing the work, it was not as a contribution to the serious history of medicine and healing. To add to the poignancy of Cockayne's situation with regard to his reputation and to posterity, Cockayne would not want the *Leechdoms* to be the sole work for which he has received some kind of fame, and the fame only happened in later years. In many ways, he seemed to think the Old English medical/magical manuscripts revealed a childish and superstitious, if necessary, side of life in Anglo-Saxon England. He was far more interested in the philological aspects of Old English, witness his concern that the major Old English dictionary of his day be correct. We must therefore sympathize with him; anyone who offers thoughts and publications to posterity shares the same helplessness as Cockayne before the world's judgment and the inevitable passage of time. Nevertheless, Cockayne's *Leechdoms, Wortcraft, and Starcunning of Early England* will remain the starting point for all studies of Anglo-Saxon medical texts.

Oswald Cockayne, the Teacher

It remains a mystery why early biographical sources state that Cockayne was "the son of a Mr. Cockin." In fact, this listing continues in the *British Biographical Index*[19] and *Modern English Biography*, who list (Thomas)

Oswald Cockayne—born in Bath in 1807[20]—as the son of a Mr. Cockin, implying that at some point he or his father must have changed the family name to Cockayne. Elsewhere, he is listed as being the son of J. Cockayne, a clerk of Bath.[21] Cockayne always signed his name and published as O. or Oswald Cockayne, yet for some unknown reason, he is now always referred to as Thomas Oswald or T. O. Cockayne. Biographers began this tradition soon after his death, yet Cockayne himself never used the given name "Thomas." From 1824 to 1828, Cockayne attended St. John's College, Cambridge, where he earned a bachelor of arts degree and where the standard biographies say he was a "tenth wrangler," meaning he excelled at mathematics. (However, the records of St. John's have him as thirtieth Wrangler for 1828 [Venn 1922–27, 80].) He became a deacon in the Church of England on 7 April 1833. That same year, he was named Curate of Keynsham; then on 2 October 1834, he was ordained in the Diocese of Bath and Wells. For a short time thereafter, he ran a school at Keynsham Grange. Why Cockayne left the school is not known, and details about his life for the next few years are lacking. It is known that in 1835 he obtained the master of arts degree from Cambridge, which then, as now, is not an earned degree.[22]

In 1842, Cockayne obtained a position as assistant master at King's College School in London, which had opened in London's Strand District in October 1831 as a junior department to King's College of the University of London. King's College was established to fill an educational gap between the Mechanics' Institutions and Oxford and Cambridge, the latter "largely the preserves of the aristocratic and the rich."[23] It was the first school of its kind in London, but by the middle of the century, it was facing competition from numerous day schools that had been opening. Finances were precarious the entire time Cockayne taught there; a 3 percent tax on salaries was enacted for several years simply to help ensure the school's survival. The school was governed by a council, whose decisions about the school's operation and personnel matters were final. Headmasters and masters taught without contracts and had to petition to be granted pensions.

Descriptions of the physical ugliness and miserable conditions at the school in the mid-1800s are recorded in some detail in *King's College School: The First 150 Years*. Before it relocated to Wimbledon in 1897, the school had the Thames to its south, the Strand to the north, and Strand Lane to the east. It occupied the ground floor and basement rooms of Somerset House, a grand building that has been renovated; however in the mid-nineteenth century the school's accommodations there were grim indeed. In fact, the author of the hymn "Onward Christian Soldiers," Sabine Baring-Gould (1834–1924), a cleric, folklorist, and prolific author who attended the school while Cockayne was there, wrote about his alma mater:

> A more depressing set of buildings could hardly have been contrived. The College and School form the east wing of Somerset House, and were built by Smirke in 1828, fossilized ugliness. We had to descend stone stairs and pass through an iron gate in which the gas was always burning. The windows, however, did look out into the hard paved play yard, surrounded by high stone walls, in which not a blade of grass showed, and not a leaf quivered in the air. The place exercised a depressing effect upon the spirits, and the boys in the playground appeared destitute of buoyancy of life, crushed by the subterranean nature of the school and the appalling ugliness of the buildings. (*KCS*, 19–20)

The basement rooms were cold and damp in winter and hot and glaring in the summer. Overcrowding was common; the playground abounded in fights and intimidation of younger boys, behavior which continued in the unsupervised privies and caused complaints from parents. Pupils regularly broke windows of neighboring houses and went wandering into the nearby theater district, which was infamous for its loose morals. In fact, one of the school's neighbors was a bordello, and its occupants could beckon when the four hundred or so boys were on the school's playground. The area around the school was dimly lit, crowded, and noisy—Dickens was describing the London to which it belonged at this very time, and in fact his eldest son, Charley, went to King's College School for one term. He left because of a serious attack of scarlet fever.

Six days a week in this cacophonous and morose setting, Cockayne taught the Upper Fourth Class in the school's Division of Classics, Mathematics, and General Literature, whose course of instruction included Divinity: Greek, Latin, English, and French; Mathematics: arithmetic; Writing: history and geography. The Upper Sixth Class learned Hebrew as well. Cockayne's classes were on Homer, Xenophon, Cicero, and Virgil, and he taught Euclidian geometry and arithmetic.

Although Miles and Cranch described Cockayne as "a most distinguished scholar . . . and the leading philologist of his day," they also said he was "a highly idiosyncratic teacher," complaints having been lodged about him in 1864 and 1866 (*KCS*, 66). In fact, Cockayne was more than idiosyncratic—he was obviously controversial. In November of 1869, Cockayne was formally accused of talking to his class "unnecessarily of subjects which could only tend to corrupt them"[24]—by then he had been an assistant master at the school for twenty-seven years. Following the accusations, a Committee of Five, including the Principal of the College and the Headmaster of the School, investigated the matter, and as notes from the school archives reveal, several boys had said that Cockayne had made what they thought were inappropriate remarks in class, and several parents had threatened to withdraw their sons if Cockayne remained their teacher. Cockayne was summoned before a subcommittee on 15 November, and the statements about his conduct were read to him to confirm or deny. The seasoned school master did not deny that he had said much of what was alleged, but in his defense, said it was far better to speak openly of such things so the boys would "have the evil effects of vice clearly set before them." Subsequently, the subcommittee withdrew a few of the statements, but left most standing, and then submitted a report to the full committee, which voted to terminate Cockayne.

The Committee of Five called Cockayne in on 20 November, at which time they dismissed him. Suddenly, he was unemployed and without any hope of finding either a scholarly or clerical appointment because he had no recommendation from the place where he had taught most of his life. Cockayne must have sensed what the outcome of the investigation would be, because he printed the small pamphlet titled "Mr. Cockayne's Narrative" that very day. In it, he stated that one person ("a Delator") made the accusations against him, that he was never given a copy of the evidence against him, and that the boys mentioned had been in his class as much as five years earlier. Even the Committee was embarrassed by the flimsiness of its own evidence, he said, adding, "The chairman of the committee, with sarcastic generosity, offered me, not the evidence, but the report seasoned to his own taste, and said I might publish it in the 'Times'."[25]

Miles and Cranch print portions of the "Narrative," some of which read as follows (the allegations, here called statements, were numbered, and Cockayne replied to them in turn):

> [It was alleged] 1. That I said Chloe was a prostitute. I reply that is not a favourite word of mine; perhaps "courtesan." 2. [That I said] "Her full time was come." That I said. What full time? answer, "Nine months." Nothing further. . . . 5. A boy had an awkward way of driving his hands down into his pockets: that I [Cockayne] said——meeting him "on the other side of the street" (so) would fancy something was the matter with him. In the place of the blank [the word that was omitted] Ladies was read. My reply: that the boy's position was offensive to the eyes, and whether I said Ladies I cannot tell after so great lapse of time. (Miles and Cranch, 66–67)

To Cockayne's printed version of the "Narrative," he appended ten letters of sympathy and support from parents and former pupils. Obviously, Cockayne had sent them the "Narrative" to elicit support, but it was to no avail. It might be added that most of the allegations against Cockayne concern discussion of incidents in classical history and mythology that involve sex, a subject that was taboo in Victorian England. The style of the reply is typical of Cockayne.

Cockayne's frank reply to statements 7 and 8 is in the records of the school and reveals more of his rather odd personal convictions.

> That I had spoken of diseases coming upon fornicators, and had alleged that
> no exemption attaches to bad women riding in carriages. Reply: that we had
> Horatius before us, a free liver, a pig of the herd of Epicurus, with his Chloes
> and Lydias and Barines, a fresh name at every ode, giving an autobiography
> of his amours, it was desirable, speaking to lads mostly of fifteen, sixteen,
> and seventeen, to warn them that his sin is visibly punished by God. Espe-
> cially that by a direct providential interference about the year 1500 A.D., God
> seeing men vicious in this respect, notwithstanding the teachings of religion,
> had sent a heavy plague to deter them. ("Narrative," 3)

In closing the "Narrative," Cockayne claimed that the Council had "declared war, especially against the age of sixty-five, at which their workers must retire pensionless." School records in fact indicate that in increasingly difficult financial times, the school let senior men go and replaced them with junior faculty, frustrating the juniors who had no hope of advancement, and forcing senior men to try to obtain positions elsewhere when they saw (or thought they saw) the handwriting on the wall.

In addition to teaching all week, Cockayne is listed as one of four masters who took students as boarders, a way many school masters of the time earned much needed extra money. He lived at 16 Montague Street in Russell Square the entire time he taught at the school. In 1865, the school's first and long-time headmaster, under whom Cockayne had taught since he entered the school, was forced to leave, but was given a pension. In that year, salaries were reduced by 3 percent, and there was growing uneasiness about the school because of its physical condition and the difficulties under which students had to study, the notorious lack of discipline, and complaints about the staff. In any case, Cockayne was immediately replaced by the Council secretary's son. Ironically, Richard Morris, the early-English scholar and philologist, was hired as First Form Master that same year.[26] The winter of 1869–70 looked bleak indeed for Oswald Cockayne.

Cockayne's Pupils: W. W. Skeat and Henry Sweet

Cockayne had another life while he was teaching boys classical languages and mathematics at King's College School—he was copying Anglo-Saxon manuscripts by hand, by the light of a candle or lantern, consulting with a number of persons on the details of what he was reading. He also kept a set of closely written notebooks that contain information about many of the texts he consulted as well as his thoughts about philological works (some of which, as mentioned, are at Houghton Library). It happened that Cockayne had two famous early English scholars as students in his classes—W. W. Skeat and Henry Sweet—but separated in time by about ten years.

Skeat was in Cockayne's Fourth Form in the early 1850s; later, in a book of reminiscences, Skeat wrote:

During part of the time when I was at King's College School, in the Strand, it was my singular fate to have for my class-master the Rev. Oswald Cockayne, well known to students as a careful and excellent Anglo-Saxon scholar, perhaps one of the best of his own date. He was an excellent and painstaking teacher, and it was, I believe, from him that I imbibed the notion of what is known as scholarship. In after life, it was my good fortune to know him personally, and I always experienced from him the greatest kindness and readiness to help. After his death, I acquired some of his books, including his well-known and useful work intitled *Anglo-Saxon Leechdoms*, and some of his carefully executed transcripts. His transcript of Ælfric's *Lives of the Saints*, in particular, has often proved useful.[27]

It may be that Skeat sold these books either to a dealer or to Medlicott (from whom Harvard obtained them), because some of the books he mentions are at Harvard.

Skeat's kind words about what he learned from his teacher did not apply to his learning Old English from Cockayne, who never taught Anglo-Saxon at the school, except perhaps informally. The painstaking work of editing, translating, and printing Anglo-Saxon manuscripts was entirely on his own time. Skeat also mentioned here that Cockayne sent him a copy of *The Shrine*, noting it abruptly breaks off at page 208, and saying he was not aware it ever went any further. He called the publication very characteristic of Cockayne and said he found the corrections to Bosworth's Anglo-Saxon dictionary published in it of service (too late, however, to be of any service to Cockayne in the 1864 encounter with Bosworth).[28] Apparently, Skeat did not keep in touch with Cockayne after he left King's College School, and it was only some years later that the two met again, in the late 1860s or early 1870s, most probably after the dismissal. Lacking academic credentials, Cockayne may well have been forced to rely on Skeat and other acquaintances for information about the manuscripts to which he earlier had easy access, and Skeat mentioned consulting some Cambridge manuscripts for Cockayne during this period.

On a personal note, Skeat told of hearing Cockayne preach:

It was once my fortune to hear Mr. Cockayne preach a sermon without notes, and I was much struck with his eloquence of expression. His language had the classic elegance of the well-read scholar, and approached more nearly the style of Johnson than I should have expected. He told me that he preferred to preach extempore, as he disliked the labour of writing down the discourse; and there was certainly no need for him to do so. (Pastime, lxvi)

The other well-known early English scholar in Cockayne's classes (1862–63) was Henry Sweet, who entered the school in 1860 and left in 1863 to study in Heidelberg. Later events connect Cockayne and Sweet over the years in a relationship that is interesting, if unclear.[29] They shared lives of professional and personal disappointments that are remarkably similar in their details, although at least Sweet was recognized in his own time as an authority on Anglo-Saxon, a recognition denied Cockayne. Miles and Cranch said in their discussion of Cockayne at King's College School (without giving a source): "Sweet, who was an eccentric in many ways, always boasted that he was self-educated, but he clearly kept in touch with Cockayne in later years, and the two reviewed each other's philological books" (*KCS*, 28). MacMahon too believes that Sweet was often in contact with Cockayne, noting that Sweet sent Cockayne a review copy of his now famous paper on the Old English dental fricatives, read to the Philological Society in 1869. At that time, Sweet was still an Oxford undergraduate and Cockayne was no longer a member of the society.

In the paper, Sweet quoted Cockayne to the effect that the letter *þ* was a late introduction in writing Anglo-Saxon, and that the oldest manuscripts used *ð* in all cases. Sweet countered Cockayne in his paper, saying the *þ* was "not altogether unknown to these early scribes."[30] In addressing Cockayne's reviewer's remarks, Sweet included Cockayne's justification for what he had written in the review—what Cockayne really meant to say by *ð* being used "in all cases" was that it was used in all grammatical cases and not "in all instances" in the early manuscripts. At the very end of Cockayne's review, referring to Sweet's explanation of how scribes used to writing Latin might have developed the *ð*, then the *þ* for writing Anglo-Saxon, Cockayne wrote: "I hope that he [Sweet] has not confused the ancient days of the Lindisfarne Latin text, with the much later time, variously placed, of the Saxon glosses" (Sweet, 184). Though outside the scope of this study, Cockayne's hard-to-follow ideas on language change and phonetics seem to be remarkably similar to those of Sweet as articulated in this early paper, where, in arguing strongly against such theories as Grimm's laws of language change, Sweet wrote, "Grimm's law has been compared to a rolling wheel; it has been described as a primary and mysterious principle, like heat or electricity; but I am unable to see in it anything but an aggregation of purely physiological changes, not necessarily connected together" (Sweet, 176). It is interesting that Sweet's professional life was later devoted to trying to distance Anglo-Saxon studies from the Germanic school of comparative philology (or linguistics) and that it most certainly was Sweet who answered Cockayne's cry to teach young students about Old English.[31] Might he have gotten at least the germ of these ideas from his schoolmaster?

Three years after delivering the paper, in 1872 when Cockayne was by now unemployed, Sweet published an unflattering review of Cockayne and Edmund Brock's *Liflade of St. Juliana* (1872) in which he wrote:

> The translations are on the whole very accurate but some of the renderings require criticism. . . . In many parts of his version Mr. Cockayne has fallen into the common error of confounding translation with transliteration. . . . This style of translation not only makes the old language ridiculous, but also exercises an injurious influence on English scholarship, by deadening the modern reader's perception of the changes (often very delicate) of meaning which many old words preserved in the present English have undergone.[32]

Such criticism from a much younger colleague (Sweet had not yet graduated from Oxford) must have hurt, and is particularly poignant when we know the strained circumstances of Cockayne's existence at the time.

If Cockayne had whetted Sweet's interest in Anglo-Saxon studies, which seems probable (under the circumstances of their knowing each other at the school), Sweet never acknowledged it. In fact, Sweet scholar M. K. C. MacMahon believes that Sweet seemed to be going out of his way to distance himself completely from Cockayne, noting an account of Sweet's academic relationship to Cockayne by Henry Cecil Wyld, a good friend of Sweet's:

> He [Sweet] received his early education from various private schools and finally at King's College School, where he was under the ferrule of Cockayne, the editor of the Leechdoms. One is tempted at first sight to relate the circumstances to the bent which Sweet's interests began to take about this time, and which was to be the ruling motive of his life. But his connection with Cockayne, purely fortuitous in origin, does not seem to have been responsible for his beginning the study of Old English, nor indeed did the afore-mentioned scholar exercise any lasting or characteristic influence upon his pupil.[33]

MacMahon believes that Wyld got this information from Sweet himself, who also said that his knowledge of Old English came from Edward Johnston Vernon's *A Guide to the Anglo-Saxon Tongue* of 1863. That there was no 1863 edition of this work, in the opinion of MacMahon, makes it even more likely that Sweet may have known the Vernon from Cockayne (editions appeared in 1846, 50, 55, 61, 65, 72, and 1878).[34]

Why Sweet (and possibly others) distanced himself from Cockayne may lie in whatever reasons there were for denying Cockayne the honorary philological position in 1861, and certainly for Sweet because of Cockayne's earlier altercation with Bosworth over the *Anglo-Saxon Dictionary*. Sweet was a rising star at Oxford and was very much in Bosworth's favor during the time Cockayne was alienating himself from the Oxford scholars. Certain other details about Sweet's life and career deserve mention because they are related to the Bosworth incident and may well have added to the unhappiness of Cockayne's last few years. MacMahon mentioned that Sweet's work on the *Student's Dictionary of Anglo-Saxon* began during his teenage years (MacMahon, 167). At the time he left King's College School and went to Heidelberg, Sweet was eighteen. It cannot be proved that Cockayne had anything to do with Sweet's dictionary, but it seems probable that he did. We know from Skeat's *Student's Pastime* that at this very time Cockayne, too, was working on an Anglo-Saxon dictionary: "At the time of his death, he had actually completed, on clearly written slips, the letters A to E [of a new Anglo-Saxon dictionary, because he was dissatisfied with Bosworth's]; and these came into my hands with the other papers" (*Pastime*, viii–ix). In the same article, Skeat said that he passed Cockayne's notes for a new Anglo-Saxon dictionary on to Professor T. Northcote Toller to use in his supplement to Bosworth. A little too late to help Cockayne were Skeat's words about Bosworth's dictionary, which Skeat said was "only a translation of Lye and Manning."

Sweet returned to England after Heidelberg, and in 1868–69 enrolled at Oxford, where Professor Bosworth taught. As Hal Momma noted, even before he entered the university, Sweet was asked to work on a revision of the Old English dictionary, an offer he declined (Momma, 2). This was precisely at the time Cockayne lost his position at King's College School and was struggling to make a living, and publishing *The Shrine*. Surely Cockayne must have known about the request for Sweet to help on the same dictionary that he had so vocally opposed only a few years earlier, and as Skeat noted, Cockayne was compiling his own entries for a new dictionary at that very time. Indeed, on the last page of *The Shrine* is a list of publications by Oswald Cockayne. It lists "A Dictionary of þe Oldest English Vulgarly Misnamed Anglo-Saxon" and "A Grammar of Saxon English" as being "in hand," but they seem never to have been published. Of the dictionary, a statement reads "From þe printed literature, and from a body of transcripts of what remains unpublished, is in preparation. Some progress has been made for þe press."

Sweet paid Cockayne at least one small compliment. In a footnote to the preface of his edition of the *Pastoral Care*, Sweet said Cockayne was the only editor in England or abroad who "did not ignore the genuine West-Saxon manuscripts" in studying King Alfred's language, others preferring "garbled reflections" (Sweet, *Alfred*, v). But the very next year, Sweet published the unflattering review of Cockayne's *Juliana* (1872), then graduated from Oxford in 1873, the year and the season in which Cockayne died, allegedly by his own hand. As Cockayne sank further into oblivion and finally into despair, Sweet's career seemed to be rapidly rising, and it appears likely that Cockayne must have known about Sweet's success in the field to which he had contributed so much, gaining little apparent reward. Yet like Bosworth and Cockayne, Sweet was studying classics at Oxford, not Germanic languages, so that he would have a better chance for a teaching position. About Sweet's early success with Anglo-Saxon, MacMahon wrote:

> By the time he [Sweet] graduated B.A. in 1873, he had already published
> the *Cura Pastoralis*, critically reviewed nine works in the academic press
> (including ones by Alexander John Ellis, John Earls, [Cockayne] and various continental philologists), read three papers to the Philological Society,
> and published three other brief items on linguistic topics. (MacMahon, 168)

It would be most interesting to know more about the nature of Cockayne's relationship with Sweet during and after King's College School.

The Final Years

After his abrupt dismissal from King's College School in November 1869, with no pension and little hope of employment, Cockayne continued to try to sell his writings. In 1870, *The Shrine* was listed as available by subscription at twenty shillings (or one shilling an issue) from the author, who had evidently moved from Montague Street to 13 Manor Park, Lee, S.E., London. He may have sold part of his personal library to raise funds. Glued into Cockayne's copy of Benjamin Thorpe's 1842 *Codex Exoniensis: A Collection of Anglo-Saxon Poetry, from a MS in the Library of the Dean and Chapter of Exeter*, which Harvard owns, at page 355 is a scrap of paper (with notes on Anglo-Saxon handwritten on the reverse). On it is a note from Trübner and Co., American Continental and Oriental Literary Agency, 60 Paternoster Row, London, dated May 10, 1872. It reads, "Mr Trübner presents his compliments to Mr Cockayne and will have much pleasure in looking at Mr Cockayne's collection any day next week. Mr Trübner will be in every day between 12 and 2 o'clock."

Thorpe's *Codex Exoniensis* was in the collection that Medlicott eventually purchased, a collection including annotated copies of Benjamin Thorpe's *Beowulf*, Bosworth's *Compendious Dictionary* of 1855, Cockayne's personal copies of his own publications, as well as several other books mentioned here. Four volumes of Cockayne's handwritten notebooks might also have been part of the collection, because they too went to Medlicott; three of them contain a miscellany of information on Anglo-Saxon, and one, as previously mentioned, contains numerous corrections to Douglas's Middle Scots translation of the *Aeneid*.[35] If he did sell—or even had to consider selling—the books that had been so much a part of his life, as witnessed by his extensive annotations in them, it must surely have added to the distress that his dismissal caused him.

Another bit of evidence as to Cockayne's strained circumstances remains in one of the handwritten notebooks at Houghton Library. On the back of hand-numbered page 330, and facing page 331, is about a third of a sheet of printed blue paper with some of Cockayne's notes on the Anglo-Saxon poem *Waldere* written on the back. The paper is from the North Western Railway of Montevideo Company, Limited, indicating that the company was founded to put in 110 miles of railway in Uruguay along the frontier with Brazil from Salto to Santa Rosa and claiming that a decree of the government from 12 December 1870 "guarantees to the Company a certain amount of revenue for 40 years from the date of opening of each section of the Line."[36] On the back of page 331 of the notebook is the rest of the blue paper, and it is dated 14 June 1872 with an offer to invest, rewards guaranteed based on the success of a similar railway in Brazil. The printed offer is signed by J. B. Davison, secretary of the Company, 113 Cannon Street. Whether Cockayne actually made an investment in the company is not known, yet the fact that he kept the paper is intriguing and points to his at least having looked into it, perhaps as a way to try to find money on which to live.

Other than these few clues, little is known about Cockayne's life after he left King's College School. In February 1998, MacMahon wrote that he had found "absolutely no reference to Cockayne in the philological literature of the 1870s. For whatever reason or reasons, he simply slid from view. Even Furnivall, that gregarious character of the Philological Society—and many others—seems to have overlooked him."[37]

Cockayne's final three years on earth were unhappy, to say the least. His efforts as a teacher and scholar of Anglo-Saxon philology had not earned him a place either as a pensioned schoolmaster or as one of the recognized experts in his chosen field. Sometime in May 1873, Cockayne went to Hastings, and in early June, his steps turned west toward the sea and Cornwall. Because at that time there was not yet a train to his destination in St. Ives, he must have gone by carriage. On the nearby cliffs in the late afternoon of June 3 or 4, Oswald Cockayne apparently took his own life. The brutal facts of what seem to be his suicide cannot be better given than by quoting in full what appeared in the *Cornish Telegraph*; the first entry is dated 18 June 1873.

Discovery of the Body of a Traveller Who Had Committed Suicide a Fortnight Since.

The greatest possible excitement was created in the town on Sunday afternoon by a report that the dead body of a man had been discovered by some children near the edge of cliffs, a little to the westward of Cardew, and which proved to be true. The same children had seen the body there a week before, and supposing it to be a man sleeping, had thrown some small pebbles to awake him and then ran away. The body was identified as that of a traveller, who had put up for a short time, about a fortnight since, at Hodge's "Western" hotel, where he had left his carpet-bag, and which remained there unclaimed. A pistol was found in his breast-coat pocket, with which he had shot himself. The body was rapidly becoming decomposed by the fortnight's exposure, and appeared to be that of a man between 50 and 60 years of age.

The man was lying on his side, with his head under a rock, and was seen there a week ago by other boys, who also thought him asleep. The boys, on Sunday, at once gave notice to P. C. Bennett, who was soon on the spot, and on turning over the body, it was found that the man had been shot through the eye, from which worms were now crawling. The ball had passed out at the back of the head, and the body was quite black from being so long dead. The only articles found in the pockets of the deceased were a map of Cornwall, a lock of hair (of a light colour,) a pistol in his coat pocket, and a powder and shot flask. The pistol had been fired off, the cap being split.

There were also 6s 10 1/2d in money, and the wearing apparel consisted of an overcoat, a black coat, vest, striped trowsers, boots with cloth tops, drawers, and stockings. Deceased is supposed to be a man about 60 years of age. He had grey whiskers, and was about 6 feet high, but it is not yet known who he was. He arrived at the "Western" hotel, on Sunday fortnight, and left the hotel on the Monday afternoon, between 3 and 4 o'clock. After paying his bill he had 6s 10 1/2d in change. He said he was only going on the hills to see the sea. Deceased left a carpet-bag at the hotel, locked.

[Below, from the *Cornish Telegraph*, Wednesday, 25 June 1873, page number not identified in the copy.]

Identification of the Gentleman Supposed to Have Committed Suicide at St. Ives.

The identity of the gentleman who was discovered dead in the neighbourhood of St. Ives, some days ago, has at last been established. On Friday the police officer at St. Ives received a telegram from a gentleman asking for information relative to the deceased's description. The reply induced the gentleman to visit St. Ives on Saturday, when he was enabled, without hesitation, to identify the deceased, from the description given and from his clothes—his body having been previously buried.

It appears that the deceased was the Rev. Thomas Oswald Cockayne, a clergyman of the Church of England, without charge, aged 65 years. He left his home, near Bristol, some weeks ago, with the avowed intention of going to Hastings, for the benefit of his health. About a week before the fatal occurrence his relatives were shocked to receive a letter from him, bearing a Western postmark; and that stating that he should never return home again. Their suspicions and fears were at once aroused, and they instituted a searching but fruitless inquiry after him. Newspaper paragraphs, announcing the sad occurrence, arrested their attention, and induced them to extend their inquiries to St. Ives, which ultimately led to the discovery of deceased.

Deceased appears to have been of an eccentric disposition, and latterly shewed unmistakable signs of melancholy. Many years ago [in fact less than three] he was one of the masters of King's College School, London, and singularly enough the Rev. J. B. Jones, vicar of St. Ives, on whom devolved the duty of paying the last sad rites to deceased, was one of his pupils at King's College at that time. Mr. Cockayne was at one time a student at St. John's College, Cambridge, where he became wrangler and B.A. in 1828, and M.A. in 1834. He entered holy orders in 1831, when he become [sic] curate of Keynsham, and was ordained priest by the Bishop of Bath and Wells in 1833.

The deceased was a man of considerable literary attainments, and had published several works, principally relating to Anglo-Saxon literature. Of these three were published in the transactions of the Philological Society, viz., "Saxon Narratiunculum," "Saxon Leechdom," and "St. Margaret, in Old English." He was also the author of a Greek syntax, a life of Turenne, and outlines of Jewish, French, and Irish histories.

In keeping with the mysteriousness of his death, no death certificate has yet been found, nor was an inquest made into the death on the cliffs. If it seems improbable that he could have shot himself through the head and then returned the weapon to an inside pocket, it does not appear to have raised a question in the mind of the authorities at that time. Why he was in St. Ives with a map—as though he were unfamiliar with the area and needed to find a certain place, perhaps to meet someone—remains an open question. No other mention of his passing, either in the form of a eulogy or even a notice, has been found other than brief newspaper obituaries though he knew and was known to the circle of Anglo-Saxonists in England and the United States at that time. In fact, the obituary column in the London *Times* for 25 June 1873 says only "At St. Ives, Cornwall, suddenly, the Rev. T. Oswald Cockayne, of Manor Park, Lee, Kent." It seems odd that the Rev. John Balmer Jones, Cockayne's pupil, did not recognize the unidentified suicide he buried at St. Ives.

The disappointments of Oswald Cockayne continue after death. He is known by a name (Thomas Oswald) he never used, and for a work (*Leechdoms, Starcraft, and Wortcunning of Early England*) he probably did not value as highly as *Spoon and Sparrow* or *The Shrine*. His life is now relegated to terse descriptions generally including the epitaph "eminent," which he did not enjoy in life. Like the former pupil who did not recognize him, posterity has buried the real Oswald Cockayne. What remains is the epitaph, "eminent scholar," which sadly misses the mark in describing this man.

Cockayne's Legacy in *Leechdoms, Wortcunning, and Starcraft of Early England*

In 1857, the British Treasury funded the Master of the Rolls to publish "materials for the History of this Country from the Invasion of the Romans to the Reign of Henry VIII" under competent editors, "preference being given, in the first instance, to such materials as were most scarce and valuable" (Cockayne 1965, 1:3). The Rolls Series is titled *Rerum Britannicarum Medii Aevi Scriptores: The Chronicles and Memorials of Great Britain and Ireland During the Middle Ages*. As mentioned, Cockayne's *Leechdoms, Wortcun-*

ning, and Starcraft of Early England began to appear in 1864 with the descriptor added to the title page "A Collection of Documents, for the Most Part Never Before Printed, Illustrating the History of Science in this Country Before the Norman Conquest."

At present, it can only be surmised how, when, and why Cockayne became interested in the Anglo-Saxon medical (or scientific) manuscripts, many of which were housed at the British Museum not far from where he lived and taught. Whether he was requested to read these particular manuscripts or did it as a matter of his own interest is not known. What Cockayne published in volume 1 was a transcription of an Anglo-Saxon translation of the *Herbarium of Pseudo-Apuleius*, a long-lived Latin medical treatise that was widely disseminated throughout Europe from the fifth century until well into the Renaissance, with his own archaic modern English translation on facing pages. The Rolls Series volumes began a new life for this ancient work (and for the other medical texts in Cockayne's volumes as well), a life largely shaped by their nineteenth-century discoverer and interpreter, who was very much a man of his time. The Latin *Herbarium of Pseudo-Apuleius* was a late-classical/early-medieval *medical* text that circulated on the continent and came to the British Isles, where it was used in Latin and in the vernacular translation. Thanks to Cockayne and the Anglo-Saxon enthusiasts of his time, the work became transformed in the mid-nineteenth century into a literary curiosity that would be studied for reasons other than medical history for many years after.

What is not generally mentioned about the *Old English Herbarium*, as the *Herbarium of Pseudo-Apuleius* became known following Cockayne's edition, is that the *Herbarium of Pseudo-Apuleius* circulated in Latin throughout the medieval West because it was a standard reference text on medicinal plants and health remedies, being copied, excerpted, quoted, and finally, translated into vernaculars. Although it ceased to be used as a work unto itself at some undetermined point, it lived on—indeed lives on—in other works that borrowed its information and used it again and again. The history of the *Herbarium of Pseudo-Apuleius*—a *medical* work—is fairly clear, a translation into Anglo-Saxon being one part of its long life (as discussed here in chapter 3). However, as a resurrected philological and cultural oddity, the *Herbarium* of Cockayne's *Leechdoms* has another story indeed.

The destiny of this once-esteemed medieval medical text was to fall into the hands of a nineteenth-century Anglo-Saxonist with peculiar attitudes toward history and linguistics, prudish concerns for morality, and biased opinions toward medicine (but as reviewed here, he lived in a time when medicine was primitive by modern standards). Oswald Cockayne had a thorough scholarly knowledge of Anglo-Saxon and a thoroughly dense scholarly approach toward translations of that language, and he elected to translate the ancient medical work and to put it in context in a series of prefaces. In 1864 the *Herbarium of Pseudo-Apuleius* emerged from the oblivion of museum storage—but as a different work, a literary creation. The following chapter discusses the *Herbarium* and its fate after being lifted from the oblivion of manuscript archives and translated into Wardour Street English, then published with prefaces destined—together with the style of translation—to prejudice the reception of this work.

Notes

1. Rev. Oswald Cockayne, ed., *Leechdoms, Wortcunning, and Starcraft of Early England*, 3 vols., Rolls Series, vol. 35 (1864–66; London: Kraus Reprint Ltd., 1965), hereafter cited in text as Cockayne 1965. Charles Singer removed Cockayne's prefaces, substituted his own preface, and reprinted this work as the Rev. Thomas Oswald Cockayne, ed., *Leechdoms, Wortcunning, and Starcraft of Early England* (London: The Holland Press, 1961); hereafter cited in text as Cockayne 1961.

2. For detailed information about the Medlicott collection and how much of it came to the Harvard libraries, see J. R. Hall, "William G. Medlicott (1816–83): An American Book Collector and His Collection," *Harvard Library Bulletin*, n.s., 1:1 (Spring 1990): 13–46. Hall's article gives the particulars of when Harvard purchased Cockayne's works from the Medlicott collection.

3. The Rev. O. Cockayne, *The Civil History of the Jews from Joshua to Hadrian; With a Preliminary Chapter on the Mosaic History* (London: John W. Parker, West Strand, 1845), 20.

4. This curious selection of works in Old English and Latin has as its full title *Narratiunculae Anglice Conscriptae: De Pergamenis Exscribebat Notis Illustrabat Eruditis Copiam* (Soho Square [London]: Iohannem R. Smith, 1861). The title page, introduction, contents page, and notes to *Narratiunculae* are all in Latin. Cockayne here transcribes the Old English and gives notes in Latin for *The Letter of Alexander to Aristotle* from Cotton Vitellius A.xv, *The Wonders of the East* from Cotton Vitellius A.xv and from Cotton Tiberius B.v, *The Passion of the Virgin-Saint Margaret* from Cotton Tiberius A.iii, excerpts from *On the Generation of Man* from Cotton Tiberius A.iii, and *Mambres Magicus* from Cotton Tiberius BV folio 87. On the inside back cover of his *Spoon and Sparrow* is the notice that "of *Narratiunculae* only 250 printed: and a right to raise the price of the last-sold copies will be reserved."

5. O. Cockayne, *The Shrine: A Collection of Occasional Papers on Dry Subjects* (London: Williams and Northgate, 1870); hereafter cited in text as *Shrine*. When these papers originally appeared is not clear, but in 1870, they were listed as available from the author by subscription at 13 Manor Park, Lee, S.E., London, the address the *Times* gave for him in its obituary of 1873. Many of Cockayne's notes for this work and for the *Narratiunculae* are in two notebooks housed at Harvard's Houghton Library, which are not dated, but have entries that Cockayne dated in 1859 through 1864.

6. Linguistics in the early-to-mid-nineteenth century is a vast topic covered in general works such as W. F. Bolton, *A Living Language: The History and Structure of English* (New York: Random House, 1982) or Thomas Pyles, *The*

Origins and Development of the English Language (New York: Harcourt, Brace, Jovanovich, 1971). Seminal works that launched the linguistic debate include Rasmus Rask's prize-winning essay on the origin of Old Norse (1818) and Jacob Grimm's *Deutsche Grammatik* (1822).

7. O. Cockayne, *Spoon and Sparrow, ΣΠΕΝΔΕΙΝ AND ΨΑΡ, FUNDERE AND PASSER; or, English Roots in the Greek, Latin, and Hebrew: Being a consideration of the Affinities of the Old English, Anglo-Saxon, or Teutonic Portion of our Tongue to the Latin and Greek; with a few pages on the Relation of the Hebrew to the European Languages* (London: Parker, Son, and Bourn, 1861); hereafter cited in text as *Spoon*.

8. Cockayne's lack of capitalization and commas has been retained in all quotes. Though a connection between the two men cannot be established, Cockayne's lack of attribution being what it is, Cockayne's ideas and muddled explanations of linguistic occurrences were quite similar to those of John Horne Tooke (1736–1812), who attempted to trace historical changes in individual words across many languages. See for example John Horne Tooke, *Epea pteroenta, or the Diversions of Purley*, new ed., rev. and corr. with additional notes by Richard Taylor (London: Printed for Thomas Tegg, 1840). *Diversions* was originally published in 1805.

9. The Rev. J. Bosworth, *The Origin of the Germanic and Scandinavian Languages and Nations: with a Sketch of their Literature, and short chronological specimens of the Anglo-Saxon, Friesic, Flemish, Dutch, the German from the Meso-Goths to the Present Time, the Icelandic, Danish, Norwegian, and Swedish: Tracing the Progress of these Languages and their Connection with the Anglo-Saxon and the Present English* (London: Longman, Rees, Orme, Brown, and Green, 1836), 2.

10. Prof. M. K. C. MacMahon, e-mail message of February 28, 1998.

11. G. Michael C. Bott, e-mail message of June 9, 2000.

12. C. B. Thurston, *A Few Remarks in Defense of Dr. Bosworth and His Anglo-Saxon Dictionaries* (London: Macmillan, 1864); hereafter cited in text as Thurston.

13. J. R. R. Tolkien, "*Beowulf*: The Monsters and the Critics," in *The Monsters and the Critics and Other Essays*, ed. C. Tolkien (London: George Allen & Unwin, 1983), 5. Tolkien gives his source as Cockayne's *Shrine*, 4. Tolkien's point in using the quote was that if Bosworth lived in 1936, Cockayne would have been able to criticize him for not reading the works because none were available, Anglo-Saxon studies having declined so greatly by that time.

14. Bishop Gawin Douglas (c. 1474–1522) wrote original Middle Scots poetry but is best known for *The XIII Bukes of Eneados of the Famose Poete Virgill Translatet out of Latyne Verses into Scottish Metir* (ca. 1500; first printed in 1553). A new edition with a glossary was issued in 1710 and may be the edition Cockayne used, since he often referred to the glossary's entries in the notebook. Why Cockayne was studying this particular translation of Virgil is not known.

15. Joseph Bosworth, *Latin Construing: or Easy and Progressive Lessons for Classical Authors, with Rules for Translating Latin into English* (London: W. Simpkin and H. Marshall, 1824), sixth edition in 1846.

16. Joseph Bosworth, *Elements of Anglo-Saxon Grammar* (London: Richard Taylor, 1823), i.

17. Velma B. Richmond, "Historical Novels to Teach Anglo-Saxonism," in Alan J. Frantzen and John D. Niles, *Anglo-Saxonism and the Construction of Social Identity* (Gainesville: University Press of Florida, 1997), 178, writes of Turner, "Very influential was Sharon Turner's *The History of the Anglo-Saxons* (1799), which Scott identifies in the preface to *Ivanhoe* as most helpful. Turner exemplified the Romantic view of history as organically unified: '[T]he past is seen as a peculiarly national affair, as having a direct connection with the present fortunes of the nation, and as an organically intertwined and self-validating system of institutions and values'[citing A. Fleishman, *The English Historical Novel*]." Turner, incidentally, claimed that he was the first to note the significance of *Beowulf*, which he brought to the public's attention in 1805.

18. Sharon Turner, *The History of the Anglo-Saxons: Comprising the History of England from the Earliest Period to the Norman Conquest (1799–1805)*, 3 vols., 4th ed. (London: Longman, Hurst, Rees, Orme, and Brown, 1823), 1:7; hereafter cited in text as Turner.

19. MacMahon wrote in June 1998 that the archives of the *British Biographical Index* (*BBI*; based in Glasgow) have Cockayne's information filed under "Cockin," but why this is so is not clear. The *BBI* is based on the *British Biographical Archives* (*BBA*), which also has T. O. Cockayne listed under "Cockin," even though its three entries about him all refer to him as Cockayne. The explanation may be that F. Boase's *Modern English Biography* (cited as one of the sources for the *BBA*), first published in 1892, appears to have the initial reference to "Cockin" as Cockayne's given name; however Boase gave no reason for the "Cockin" reference. The *Dictionary of National Biography*, on the other hand, first published in 1917 (but founded in 1882) lists him as Thomas Oswald Cockayne, philologist, with no information about his place of birth or parents. It makes no reference to the alleged "Cockin" parentage.

20. The *BBI* lists only the year of his birth; his place of birth is listed in John Venn, *Alumni Cantabrigiensis: A Biographical List of All Known Students, Graduates and Holders of Office at the University of Cambridge from the Earliest Times to 1900*, vol. 2 (Cambridge: Cambridge University Press, 1922–27); hereafter cited as Venn. Singer in Cockayne 1961, preface to vol. 1, listed his birth date as 1809, but he provided no sources for his biographical information on Cockayne.

21. Venn, 80. MacMahon learned directly from St. John's College that the county of Cockayne's birth was Somerset, and that the College lists his father as *the Rev.* J. Cockayne (emphasis added).

22. The details of his ordination and priesthood are from Venn; only the Cambridge dates and degrees are in the *BBI*. No sources located indicate whether Cockayne was ever married. Singer in Cockayne 1961, preface to vol. 1, xvii, said Cockayne took Holy Orders in 1831 and "was later Curate of Keynsham"; he did not mention his master's degree. Singer also said that Cockayne became an assistant master at King's College School "two or three years later" (it was actually not until 1842, eight years after he was ordained and

seven after obtaining the master's degree) and said only that he taught "general subjects." Singer gave no more dates for Cockayne's life and death, although he did mention his dismissal from the school "under distressing circumstances," his apparent subsequent poverty, and death by his own hand.

23. Frank Miles and Graeme Cranch, *King's College School: The First 150 Years* (London: King's Cross School, 1979), 1; hereafter cited in text as *KCS*. Details about the school and Cockayne's tenure there are from this same book unless otherwise noted.

24. The archives of King's College provided photocopies of the allegations (or statements as they are called) about Cockayne as well as Cockayne's defense, a printed pamphlet of four pages titled "Mr. Cockayne's Narrative." In the "Narrative" is his remark that he had been "thirty three years in the service of King's College School," when in fact, the official records show him to have been an assistant master from 1842–1869 (not 1836). Perhaps he worked in a part-time capacity for the school, and this would explain what he did after leaving the school in Keynsham Grange in the mid-1830s.

25. Cockayne's remarks are quoted from Miles and Cranch and from Cockayne's privately printed pamphlet, "Mr. Cockayne's Narrative," photocopy from King's College archives, ref. IC/68, with permission of King's College School; hereafter cited in text as "Narrative." The details of the dismissal are in Miles and Cranch, 65–7.

26. Charlotte Brewer, in her chapter on Walter William Skeat in Helen Damico, ed., *Medieval Scholarship: Biographical Studies on the Formation of a Discipline* (New York: Garland Press, 1998), 139–150, says that Skeat acknowledges Morris's considerable influence on his work in Middle English. Skeat was one of Cockayne's pupils.

27. Rev. Walter W. Skeat, *A Student's Pastime: Being a Select Series of Articles Reprinted from "Notes and Queries"* (Oxford: Clarendon Press, 1896), viii; hereafter cited in text as *Pastime.*

28. Sweet too brought up the topic of Bosworth's dictionary. Although he did not say he agreed with Cockayne's personal attack on Bosworth's scholarship, he mentioned in a footnote the "highly amusing instances of the way in which gross errors have arisen and been handed down from dictionary to dictionary" that Cockayne published in *The Shrine*. See Henry Sweet, *King Alfred's West Saxon Version of Gregory's Pastoral Care* (1871; London: Kegan, Paul, Trench, Trübner, reprinted 1930), vii; hereafter cited in text as Sweet *Alfred.*

29. See M. K. C. MacMahon, biography of Henry Sweet in Helen Damico, *Medieval Scholarship*; hereafter cited in text as MacMahon.

30. Henry Sweet, "The History of the TH in English" (1869) in H. C. Wyld, *Collected Papers of Henry Sweet* (Oxford: Clarendon Press, 1913), 176; hereafter cited in text as Sweet. (First printed in the *Transactions of the Philological Society, 1868–69,* London, 272–88.)

31. Hal Momma in "Old English as a Living Language: Henry Sweet and an English School of Philology," a paper presented at the annual conference of the International Society of Anglo-Saxonists, Palermo, Sicily, Italy, July 1997; hereafter cited in text as Momma. Momma said that Sweet thought the

philology of Germany was one-sided and defective, privileging written letters over spoken sounds of living languages and dialects.

32. Henry Sweet, review of *Liflade of St Juliana, Academy* III, 52 (15 July 1872): 278. In 1871, in the preface to the *Pastoral Care* (x), Sweet was careful to point out that in his translation he "carefully avoided that heterogeneous mixture of Chaucer, Dickens, and Broad Scotch, which is affected by so many translators from the Northern languages."

33. Henry Cecil Wyld, "Henry Sweet," *Modern Language Quarterly* IV, ii (July 1901): 73.

34. Edward Johnston Vernon, *A Guide to the Anglo-Saxon Tongue: A Grammar after Erasmus Rask* (London: J. R. Smith, 1846).

35. The notebook on Douglas is catalogued as 12491.11 at Houghton Library, Harvard.

36. Houghton Library, Harvard, MS 641.1, vol. 2.

37. M. K. C. MacMahon, e-mail of February 1998. Frederick James Furnivall (1825–1910) directed the Early English Text Society publications for many years, and Cockayne published in the series.

2

Cockayne's *Herbarium*

It will be difficult for the kindliest temper to give
a friendly welcome to the medical philosophy
of the Saxon days.
—Oswald Cockayne, *Old English Herbarium*

Transformations

Several modern misconceptions about medieval medicine and magic, particularly in Anglo-Saxon England, were suggested by Cockayne's prefaces and
translations in *Leechdoms, Wortcunning, and Starcraft of Early England.*
Though he may not have intended it, he helped advance an attitude that
medieval medicine was preposterous, that intelligent people could not have
taken it seriously, and that it could not have worked much, if at all. The prej-
udicial attitude he exhibited toward early medieval medicine continues today
and is the first misconception explored here.

Also from Cockayne's prefaces emerged an image of Anglo-Saxon
leeches, as he liked to call the healers of the time, vainly seeking to compre-
hend classical remedies that were beyond their intellectual reach while chant-
ing gibberish and saying nonsensical words reflecting native magic. This
suggestion encouraged later scholars beginning with historian Charles Singer
to distinguish between the degenerating classical medicine carried on in library
texts from native medico-magic, the supposed norm in practice. The argument
presented here, by contrast, is that medicine and native (Germanic) magical
practices are nearly impossible to separate in early medieval texts, an argument
bolstered in chapter 3, where a pan-European, early medieval medical tradition
is described, which combined magic and medicine in its nascent stages.

The last misconception discussed here is the false impression Cockayne's translations leave on the reader (and left in his own day): They

emphasize the notion that the subject matter is, if not ludicrous, woefully antiquated. Far from being straightforward translations, his *Leechdoms, Wortcunning, and Starcraft* represent a transformation of ancient texts on healing into literary oddities. In all fairness, this was not Cockayne's intent; he merely wanted to emphasize their ancient Germanic origins. Unfortunately, he chose an archaizing style of translation that was in vogue among some Victorians although ridiculed by others. It is a style that perpetuates misconceptions about the material and its seriousness. This chapter discusses these continuing misunderstandings about early medieval and Anglo-Saxon medical texts, the *Old English Herbarium* in particular, that continue because of and in spite of Oswald Cockayne.

The State of Medicine in Cockayne's Time

Cockayne's prefaces to each of the three volumes of the *Leechdoms* reflect his historical perspective and his bias concerning primitive medicine. However, medicine and pharmacology during Cockayne's lifetime were in many respects closer to those of the medieval period than to those of the twentieth century. In the few places in his prefaces where Cockayne addressed medicine, and not Anglo-Saxon culture in general, it was to express horror or dismay at Anglo-Saxon practices; yet from the vantage point of modern medicine, dismay and horror are the general reactions to the nineteenth-century medicine Cockayne knew. To put his translations and prefaces in context, a brief overview of the state of medicine as Cockayne would have experienced it is in order.

Medicine was entering a new era in the second half of the nineteenth century; it might be fair to say that the long tradition of medical care that originated with the Greeks and Romans was finally ending—at least as the basis for officially sanctioned medicine as practiced in most Western countries. That long-standing medical approach was largely based on empiric remedies prescribed after observation of the patient and drawing on received wisdom about medicinal plants and minerals, used either alone or in compounds with other plants, and mixed with a variety of substances.[1] Treatment was founded more on knowledge that a remedy *seemed* to help rather than on *why* it helped, using scientific knowledge of disease and the chemistry of healing medications.

Louis Pasteur (1822–95) began to publish his pioneering discoveries in bacteriology in the 1860s, explaining how epidemics spread. Because of his writings, use of vaccinations and "pasteurization" became more widespread, and disinfectants were more common in preventing contamination and infection. At the same time Cockayne was writing about the surgical skills of the Greeks and Romans, many surgeons were just beginning to use anesthesia, and it took until the turn of the century for anesthetics to win acceptance by the majority of surgeons. (The first successful demonstration of ether was in 1846 at Massachusetts General Hospital and the use of anesthesia spread rapidly thereafter; even so, it was not universally accepted.) Needless to say, for much of Cockayne's life, surgery was a last resort for many, the patient often preferring death rather than submitting to the knife.[2] Without anesthesia, the challenges facing a surgeon in cutting into and performing a procedure on a thrashing and screaming patient were daunting. Prevention of infection and the ability to sedate patients enabled surgery to achieve tremendous advances during the late nineteenth century. It was then that surgery became a respected part of the medical profession after centuries of being looked down upon as mere barber-surgery. As Inglis noted, "The war between physicians—who thought of themselves as the only true doctors—and the surgeons had been particularly venomous," and was underway with a vengeance as early as the thirteenth century (Inglis, 133).

Life expectancy throughout Europe during Cockayne's lifetime was forty years, by 1900 it was fifty, and in 1950 it was seventy, a fact that is generally attributed to improvements in preventive medicine in the late nineteenth century and to continual improvement in nutrition.[3] But the history of medicine tends to be written in terms of famous men and milestone achievements, not in terms of mundane statistical knowledge, as Erwin Ackerknecht put it:

> The mundane character of preventive medicine has made it a stepchild in the eyes of medical history and in the sympathies of the larger public. Even in this book, the history of preventive medicine has played second fiddle to the history of clinical medicine. This is due mainly to the fact that our medical education is primarily designed to prepare clinicians who treat diseases rather than to prevent disease.[4]

Many medical historians attribute swift advances in medicine in the later nineteenth century to the Industrial Revolution with its rapidly increasing urban population and the attendant woes related to health under crowded and unsanitary conditions, a sad phenomenon that also enabled clinical observation to be made on large numbers of people and statistics to be kept on diseases, treatments, and the success with cures. (For medicine in the later nineteenth century, see Inglis, "Public Health," 165–71, and Ackerknecht, "Public Health and Professional Development in the Nineteenth Century," 195–202.)

Specialization was just coming into being in the mid-1800s when Cockayne lived, and although it is now characteristic of Western medical practice, the general practitioner and general surgeon of the time opposed it because of its traditional association with traveling quacks, as Ackerknecht discusses in his chapter 17, "The New Specialism of the Nineteenth Century." Ackerknecht also said in 1955 that more than half the physicians in the United States were specialists, with fifteen areas of specialization being recognized, whereas in the 1850s, medicine recognized only four broad areas that had existed for centuries: medicine, surgery, obstetrics, and gynecology. Not everyone, even today, applauds the increasing trend toward specialization, and Inglis laments the demise of the general physician in favor of specialists who are in "watertight compartments which too often cut off the specialist, not merely from other branches of medicine, but from wider interests" (Inglis, 144).

Part of Inglis's discussion about "The Doctor and the Quack" deals with the mostly adversarial relationship between physicians and apothecaries (in addition to their quarrels with the surgeons). Local apothecaries actually acted as general practitioners; they compounded their own prescriptions, made house visits, and were far less expensive than physicians. Speaking about the time when Cockayne lived, Inglis described apothecaries in England:

> The chief complaint about apothecaries was that they cheated the patient by prescribing bogus drugs: as they made prescriptions up themselves the temptations must often have been too much for them. . . . But in Britain, the apothecaries managed to entrench themselves as general practitioners, in spite of the powerful attacks mounted on them [by physicians and chemists]. . . . The apothecaries, however, were lucky in that they acquired status just in time to be recognized as doctors, when the various and previously disunited elements of the medical profession began to coagulate into a profession. (Inglis, 135–36)

In the United States, interestingly enough, the rural nature of much of the country tended to prolong the life of the doctor/apothecary/surgeon in one person.

A student at King's College School soon after Cockayne began teaching there (1844–45), Sabine Baring-Gould vividly remembered details of his own medical treatment as a child in the mid-nineteenth century as he penned his memoirs in 1922. Having received great relief from pleurisy when his mother applied mustard poultices to his chest, Gould's opinion toward them soon changed:

> I had them [mustard poultices] not only applied to my chest and to my back, but also on one occasion behind and below my ears. There the poultice was kept on so long that when removed it carried off my skin with it, and the fresh growth was brown as the hide of a West Indian. . . . Not only did the windows of apothecaries display in those days outspread yellow wax-bedaubed chamois leathers, but also, what was more interesting, globes full of water, containing leeches. I have on my chest to this day the triangular scars produced by the bites of those blood-suckers. . . .

> My constitution must have been robust, in spite of the opinion of the
> physicians, or I could not have survived the draughts of castor-oil, the blue
> pills followed by drenches of senna and salts, the powders barely disguising
> themselves in raspberry jam, the ipecacuanha doses, the gargles, the plas-
> ters, the blisters, the cotton-wool paddings before and behind the ribs, the
> leeches, the cuppings and the bleedings.[5]

During Cockayne's lifetime, it was not always clear exactly who was a
reputable physician and who was a quack; indeed, it would be difficult to
make such a distinction in an age predating regulation of the medical, surgical, and pharmaceutical professions. In an essay on medical ethics in the
nineteenth century, Peter Bartrip wrote:

> When referring to the early nineteenth or previous centuries there are sound
> reasons for avoiding pejoratives, for with medical training and qualification
> highly variable, it was often far from clear precisely who was the
> quack. . . . As for the medical corporations, which were supposed to regu-
> late the profession, these were, in reality, unable to prevent the unqualified
> from practising or even to warrant the skill and probity of their members.
> Thomas Wakley [an early editor of the *Lancet*], it should be remembered,
> built the reputation of the *Lancet* by exposing quackery and incompetence
> in high, as well as in low places.[6]

Bartrip showed that this situation prevailed through most of the century,
and even licensed physicians lent their names to "secret remedies and nostrums" since it was a major source of income. The ethical question then arose
as to whether the formula could be kept secret from other physicians if it
indeed promoted health, but of course the risk was that the ingredients could
either be replicated and sold by others or shown to be bogus. In turn, Bartrip
wrote, the *British Medical Journal* (which became recognized early on as the
organ of the British Medical Association) derived much of its income from
advertisements for these potions and nostrums—the question raised even at
that time was whether it was ethical to do so. Patent medicines, meaning prepared remedies sold over the counter and touted to cure one or more ailments, and medical cults outside established medicine—for example,
osteopathic and chiropractic healing, Christian Science, spiritualism, and
mesmerism—were also developing in parallel with was what happening
within the medical establishment.

Perhaps Cockayne shared the increased public interest in health issues,
shown by the number of periodicals devoted to the topic: "For various reasons, the nineteenth century saw huge growth in the number of medical jour-
nals including from 1823, weeklies which dispensed a varied diet of news,
opinion, scholarly articles and so forth" (Bartrip, 196). Chemical and medicinal preparations made up the majority of the advertisements, and the medical

literature showed that physicians were divided as to their opinion toward them. The situation sounds much the same as it is today, with hundreds of remedies readily available at local drugstores without a prescription and promising myriad cures.

Various schools of herbal medicine were legal and popular in Cockayne's lifetime, and it was not until the twentieth century that medicinal plants no longer were part of the official medical curriculum. A brief history of herbal medicine described its practice during Cockayne's time as follows:

> Like the undercurrent of hostility between Chiropractors and Osteopaths, or between herbalists and homeopaths, this in-fighting [between schools of herbal medicine] only proved the claim by regular medicine that herbalists were unscientific and their system was in disarray. Instead of joining forces, herbalists insisted on their distinct party loyalties. [Albert Isaiah] Coffin was proud, for instance, that he knew nothing of pathology, pointing out his daily habit of curing things which regular doctors claimed to understand but could not cure. [John] Skelton saw the wider issues, speaking for a complement of diverse therapies. . . . At least the various splinter groups of herbal medicine managed to deluge Parliament with protests against anti-herb legislation.[7]

Cockayne verified this state of affairs in medicine in the preface to volume 1 of the *Leechdoms*, where he wrote:

> Our own medicines are very largely taken from what we call the vegetable kingdom; but their composition is concealed from the patient by the mysteries of prescriptions and of foreign names. A sick man thinks himself effectively tended, if he chance to make out that his doses contain Taraxacum, Belladonna, Aconite, Hyoscyamus, or Arneca, or if he be refreshed with Ammonia; but he smiles contemptuously at the herb woman who administers dent de lion, nightshade, wolfsbane, henbane, elecampane, or who burns horn in the sick chamber. Perhaps herbs are more really effectual than we shall easily believe. (Cockayne 1965, 1: liii)

In brief, this was the world of healthcare Cockayne would have known while he copied out the Anglo-Saxon medical treatises toward the middle of the nineteenth century—it was a medical world that many today would not consider modern but "medieval," as often used today to mean primitive.

Cockayne's *Herbarium* and Its Influence on the Reception of Medieval Medicine

The verdict on medieval medicine since the time of Cockayne's 1864 prefaces and translations can at best be called controversial. His editions of the Anglo-Saxon medical texts—widely cited by anyone working with early medicine in England—are part of the generally negative foundation of scholarship about the topic since he wrote, a foundation that may be finally eroding. In addition, his prefaces to the three volumes of the *Leechdoms* were negative in tone toward the Anglo-Saxons and their attempts at medical treatment, and these prefaces presaged later writers.

By using selected quotations from a wide assortment of medieval medical works as Cockayne did, anyone can certainly exaggerate what moderns consider to be the ludicrous in them, and Cockayne's translations and the information contained in his prefaces have long been a major source for histories discussing early medieval medicine. Unfortunately, many later writers on the subject not only adopt Cockayne's disdain for herbal cures, incantations, charms, and the like, but extend that disdain to all of medieval medicine. The evaluation of healing practices during the Dark Ages as summarized by S. G. B. Stubbs and E. W. Bligh in *Sixty Centuries of Health and Physick* is fairly typical for general medical histories. In a chapter titled "A Thousand Years of Darkness," they wrote:

> We have chosen to attempt a brief note on the medieval background rather than to present strings of names of tedious writers and lengthy specimens of the futilities of medieval recipe books. It is obvious that if this attempt be a fair representation nothing in the way of medical science as we understand it could exist. In fact it did not—in Europe.[8]

Theirs is certainly not an isolated evaluation, and although Cockayne himself did not cause all the negativity, his translations and prefaces contributed to it.

For example, in an 1898 essay under the rubric "Odd Volumes" in which he considered several older works, the Right Honorable Sir Herbert Maxwell, Bart., M.P. turned to "a collection of Anglo-Saxon treatises on medicine," which he said were admirably edited by Cockayne.[9] Maxwell in many ways expanded on the prejudice toward medieval healing practices that Cockayne's prefaces suggested, and he was even more pointed. Maxwell wrote, for example:

> one turns indolently to it [Cockayne's work] to see what mad or blind pranks our forefathers played with their constitutions, and to thank God that we are not such blockheads as they. In truth, many of the remedies prescribed seem worse than the diseases they professed to cure: unspeakably nasty, some of them . . . (Maxwell, 660)

In this review were notions whose echoes are heard even today, such as the certainty that even the physicians and wise men of the day did not believe in the cures they prescribed and used because they were obviously ludicrous even then. Another was that the Teutonic healers vainly tried to understand classical medicine and because they could not, they simply passed on written remedies blindly without knowing why. Maxwell did not dwell on the use of magic in Anglo-Saxon medicine, though he mentioned superstition and use of prayers and pagan charms together. The outlook in the essay very much reflected Cockayne's and Sharon Turner's as discussed in the previous chapter: a benevolent consideration of the childhood of the English nation.

Even though the Celtic tradition was and is strong in large parts of Great Britain, neither Turner nor Cockayne treated it at any length, and they did not discuss a unique Celtic medical tradition that might have underlain or contributed to the Anglo-Saxon; their goal after all was to find the roots of Anglo-Saxon culture. In fact, both men expressed quite a bias against the Celts, whom they considered inferior. Turner claimed the Celts lost the moral virtue they needed to survive, in contrast to the superior Saxons who completed their destiny in laying the foundation for Great Britain (Turner, 1:196–242). Cockayne even said the Saxons were given "the Keltic careless tribes for a prey" (Cockayne 1965, 1:x).

Moreover, few modern works attempt to deal with ancient Celtic *medicine* itself, scholars preferring to study Celtic divination and magic (a trend seen in studying the Anglo-Saxon medical works as well, as discussed later). However in *Magie, médecine et divination chez les Celtes*, Christian-J. Guyonvarc'h looked closely at Celtic medicine and found that healing was part of the duties of the druids, that medicine and spiritual practices were intertwined. He said that because the druids learned everything orally in a secret twelve-year apprenticeship, nothing was written down. Thus, only remnants of the druids' healing practices may have survived the years of their being outlawed under the Roman Empire and being suppressed by Christianity. Therefore, precious little—if any—of the Celtic (druidic) healing tradition survived even into Anglo-Saxon times. Guyonvarc'h concluded:

> Nous avons quelques notions précises sur le matériel chirurgical de la Gaule romaine, mais nous ne savons absolument rien sur celui des Celtes insulaires, rien non plus sur la pharmacopée irlandaise et, tout compte fait, relativement peu de choses sur la pharmacopée celtique continentale de l'Antiquité, hormis mention des plantes, dont celle que nous connaissons le mieux, grâce à Pline l'Ancien, est le gui.[10]

In addition, Guyonvarc'h argued that medicinal plant lore must have been widespread and fairly homogeneous in the ancient world and that early medicine was probably quite similar everywhere, with everyone, including the Celtic druids, using the same basic natural ingredients.

Forty years after Cockayne's *Leechdoms* was published, in a stated effort to spark interest in the history of English medicine, Joseph Frank Payne, M.D., gave two lectures before the Royal College of Physicians in June 1903, citing "lamentable apathy and but little industry" on the part of British medical historians toward studying the history of their profession in England from the earliest time.[11] Central to his topic were the Anglo-Saxon medical texts Cockayne had translated, texts that, according to Payne, still had not received the attention they deserved. He told his audience that Cockayne's works presented all that was left of the medical library of Anglo-Saxon England, yet in a prefatory note to the published lectures, he acknowledged having received help from Henry Bradley, who, he said "corrected a large number of inaccuracies in Mr. Cockayne's translation of the Anglo-Saxon texts" (Payne, v). Bradley, as noted earlier, was an editor of the *Oxford English Dictionary*. Nothing more was said in the lectures or in notes in the book about Bradley's alleged corrections to Cockayne's work, and the content and extent of these corrections are not known.

Payne portrayed the tradition that the library of Anglo-Saxon medicine represented in a much more sympathetic light than Cockayne, Turner, and Maxwell. In contrast particularly to Cockayne, Payne praised the intelligence and ingenuity of the Anglo-Saxons:

> In no other European country was there, at that time or for centuries after, any scientific literature written in the vernacular. . . . This is proof that the Anglo-Saxons possessed high intelligence and activity of mind; though not necessarily that they possessed deep learning. . . . The other quality which we find in the medical as in the pure literature, and which seems characteristic of the Anglo-Saxon mind, is that readiness to learn from all sources, that hospitality to ideas, of which I have already spoken. (Payne, 33)

Payne considered *Bald's Leechbook* to be the most important of the Anglo-Saxon medical texts because it was an original compilation written in Old English using a variety of sources. He considered the *Herbarium* to be "a continuation of the noble project of that great king [Alfred], to put in the hands of his people the best books of all kinds, written in their native tongue," and later in the lecture, Payne outlined the great importance of the *Herbarium* to the early medieval world (Payne, 38). However, he observed that, not withstanding the merits of the texts, they could not transcend the time in which they were written. Echoing Cockayne, Payne described the early medieval period to be "the time when European medicine stood at its very lowest level; and if any period deserved the name of the dark ages it was this" (Payne, 57).

Yet Payne displayed a remarkably tolerant attitude for his time toward the allegedly superstitious elements of Anglo-Saxon medicine: "the charms, incantations, exorcisms, the wearing of amulets or other magical objects, the employment of ceremonies and religious rites in the gathering or preparations of medicines, and so forth" (Payne, 94). He said that what modern Englishmen would call superstition had been part of every known medical

system to the present and he characterized the modern European art of healing as an exception. In more detail than Cockayne's prefaces, and certainly
more lucidly, Payne contrasted the Greek art of healing—with its lack of
superstition or appeal to supernatural beliefs—with most other healing sys-
tems in the world, all of which have relied on various forms of superstition.

With regard to the charms and other superstitious materials in the Anglo-
Saxon medical texts, Payne, like Cockayne, touched on the possibility of
being able to trace their origin to a locale or a tribe, acknowledging that much
pagan material had very probably been adapted to the Christian pantheon as
time progressed. Payne devoted considerable space to this discussion, and it
seems obvious he was responding to a known interest in this side of the
ancient healing arts. He took the position that it was difficult, if not impossible to determine with certainty the origin of any one charm or practice, noting that they came out of a tradition spanning a great deal of time and a huge
geographic area (including countries surrounding and affecting the West), at
a time and place when superstition and healing were inextricably intertwined. Apropos this topic, Payne remarked:

> It is not easy from the form or contents of a charm to know whether it orig-
> inated in folklore or in borrowed learning. A great deal of so-called "folk-
> medicine" is old-fashioned regular medicine which has sunk down to the
> level of the unlearned, and has sometimes put on a rustic dress. It is not all
> so, of course, but many charms and the like collected by students of folklore
> and called provincial may be traced to Oriental, Greek, or Latin sources
> (Payne, 108). . . . It is probable that, if we knew more about it, we should
> find the roots of other portions in the old folk-lore of the Teutonic and
> Celtic peoples, but of this I am not competent to speak. (Payne, 142)

Many of the topics Payne discussed in 1903 were repeated almost in his
own words beginning in the 1920s by Charles Singer, whose most accessible
works do not acknowledge or cite Payne. However, if Singer appropriated
ideas from Payne, he did so with a decided agenda and gave them his own
bent. Singer's writings are numerous and ubiquitous and have long been part
of the essential readings for those who write on medieval medicine.[12] Singer,
like Payne, saw in the Old English (indeed in all medieval) medical texts a
conglomeration of traditions, one of which was the end of Greek rational
medicine, in his words "the last stage of a process that has left no legitimate
successor, a final pathological disintegration of the great system of Greek
medical thought."[13] Throughout his many works, this message resounds:
Medieval medicine is monstrous and preposterous.

As mentioned earlier, Singer reissued the three-volume *Leechdoms* in
facsimile in 1961 and substituted his own preface for Cockayne's, saying:
"Each of the three [original] volumes had a long preface. These we omit
because they are misleading in the present state of knowledge" (Cockayne

1961, 1:xx). And so in this edition of the *Leechdoms,* the bias in Singer's 1952 *Magic and Medicine* was even more closely linked to the Old English works, much of it gleaned from what Cockayne and Payne had said without crediting them with the ideas. The following was typical for Singer in evaluating medicine in Anglo-Saxon England:

> The Anglo-Saxon leech had no originality. That quality, for him, would have a negative value. He had no understanding of even the rudiments of the science of classical antiquity. His sources were very various and the demonstration of them provides the chief interest of these volumes of Cockayne. The general level of this medicine will be found far lower, far more barbarous, than the common accounts of Anglo-Saxon culture suggest. The sources of this debased material, if accurately and completely displayed, would reveal much of the social circumstances of England for several centuries before and for a century after the Conquest. . . .
>
> [T]hus Cockayne's *Leechdoms* should be regarded as an end not a beginning. They provide good examples of the darkest and deliquescent stage of a [sic] outdated culture. (Cockayne 1961, 1:xix–xx, and xlvii)

About ten years later, Wilifrid Bonser, one of Singer's pupils, continued Singer's ideas in detail in a book whose title, *The Medical Background of Anglo-Saxon England,* is misleading, and whose subtitle actually tells the truth: "A Study in History, Psychology, and Folklore." The preconceived notions about medicine and what motivated its healers that was seen in Cockayne and Singer were repeated and amplified here. Though the following statement was not attributed to Singer, it exactly carried on his ideas and perpetuated the ideas he promoted about early medieval medicine generally, Anglo-Saxon in particular:

> Western medicine stagnated for more than five hundred years from the later Imperial Roman times until it began to revive in the hands of the Arabs. The chief reason for this stagnation was the lack of that inquiring spirit to which one is accustomed today. . . . Most leeches were content to copy dead material without questioning this authority.[14]

Yet Singer's verdict on medieval medicine was not accepted unanimously in his day, even though it proved—and continues to prove—to be quite popular. Historian Loren MacKinney disagreed with Singer, his contemporary, on the question of exactly what medieval medicine represented:

> Dr. Singer, the eminent English scholar, has defended medieval medical history on the ground that it is a study in the pathology of civilization. But it is more than this; it is the birth and growth of a new civilization. Early medieval civilization consisted of two healthy elements, and one that was old and pathological. In the West, although classical civilization was sick

unto death, much of it was preserved through its union with a vigorous young religion (Christianity) and a sturdy new race of rulers (the Germans). These two furnished the active elements by which a practically new civilization was created. *The early middle age is a period in which the clergy, originally dedicated to supernatural healing, and the Germanic people, addicted to primitive folk medicine, slowly progressed to the point where they could appreciate classical medical science and apply more intelligently the results of their own practical experience* [emphasis added].[15]

MacKinney cited examples of bias such as Singer's (and carried on by Bonser) toward the "Dark Ages" in several nineteenth-century scholars, and attributed this prejudiced attitude toward the Middle Ages to received knowledge from high-school history teachers with outmoded views. He wrote, "Many an educated man's conception of the early middle ages is merely an amplified image of the term dark age, the sole remnant of youthful acquisitions in a history class" (MacKinney, 21).

Stanley Rubin, a somewhat later writer on the subject, shared MacKinney's objectivity about examining the details of medieval remedies to see if they might have helped the patient at all, but his *Medieval English Medicine* also demonstrates a personal bias similar to that in Cockayne, Singer, and Bonser against the whole tradition of medicine in Anglo-Saxon England. Rubin's work concentrates on Anglo-Saxon and the early years of Norman England, and cites interesting archaeological evidence to give substance to the narrative that few other works use. However, instead of being grounded in the concrete, the work is replete with assumptions prefaced by words like "undoubtedly" and "no doubt" and postulations of what might have been.

Rubin repeatedly underscored the terrible living conditions that must have prevailed at the time, but not from an objective archaeologist's point of view. For example, with no citation of sources, he described the miserable dwellings of the early Anglo-Saxons as being semisunken and stated, again without archaeological or other evidence: "Refuse would quickly accumulate and general squalor prevailed."[16] He continued in the same passage: "Domestic hygiene was impossible under these conditions and infectious diseases and others caused by squalor and dirt would have been common and widespread." The evidence now available for living conditions and medical treatment in Anglo-Saxon England certainly does not put the Anglo-Saxons on a level high enough to satisfy the sanitary concerns of the twentieth-century Western world, but "squalor" is not a term to be used lightly. If Rubin had cited as much archaeological data for all of his descriptions of life in Anglo-Saxon England as he did for diseases shown in skeletal remains, his picture would have much more validity. The way of life then may have been primitive by our standards, but substantive evidence would show just how primitive it actually was and whether there were any redeeming features. In their dissertations on Anglo-Saxon medical works, Barbara Olds and Frieda Hankins adopted Rubin's technique of reaching a number of "doubtless" conclusions, and they both cited Rubin's work.[17]

In discussing Rubin's book, an apparently offhand remark concerning Cockayne must be mentioned. In light of his actual place among Anglo-Saxonists, it could be seen as cruel: "In this monumental work a modern English translation of much of this material is presented, and while in some instances the translation may not meet the demands of more recent standards of scholarship, this does not in any way detract from the success the editor undoubtedly achieved" (Rubin, 44). The unhappy life and lack of success of Cockayne are discussed in chapter 1. In leaving Rubin, a final quote is in order, summing up in many ways the author's biases toward the tradition as a whole yet objectivity toward some of the details: "While much of what is to be discussed in this and other chapters may seem crude, distasteful in parts and perhaps even useless from a modern medical point of view, it was, at least, the serious and not ignoble attempt of an early population to alleviate suffering and distress—a not unworthy endeavor" (Rubin, 45). A new way of looking at medieval medical practices that is at variance with the above-mentioned scholars is presented in chapter 3. This approach, shaped by researchers such as Linda Voigts, John Riddle, and M. L. Cameron, compares medieval practices with the very similar and very old traditions of herbology and *curanderismo* (folk medicine in Hispanic culture).

If Cockayne's condescending attitude toward medieval medicine has persisted into the present, fueled to some extent by Singer's legacy, so has his implied distinction between native and classical medical practices, a distinction that has also promoted serious misconceptions about the state of medicine in Anglo-Saxon England and early medieval Europe generally. Cockayne compared Anglo-Saxon medical practices and knowledge unfavorably to the Greek and Roman, even saying Anglo-Saxon leeches lacked the intellectual power to understand classical medicine. He also wrote at length about the Anglo-Saxons' superstitions and charms and other primitive practices, which he believed they brought with them when they migrated into England. Cockayne simply made this distinction in his prefaces based on what he surmised he knew from the texts and his own understanding of history; it has subsequently become received wisdom.

The modern literary/historical custom has been to categorize late classical and medieval medical texts as being primarily from the rational Greek tradition or from the barbaric and superstitious one. This neat division has been especially prevalent in Anglo-Saxon studies, and if Cockayne did not invent it, his writings certainly contributed to its becoming established as fact—primarily by Singer and Bonser, who espoused it vocally and spent much energy in identifying the origins of separate (largely) folkloric aspects of medicine/magic. However, this division of types is more suited to literary studies than to medical history. It does not appear to reflect correctly what was going on in a tradition of healing that used a fluid body of texts, oral transmission, and a system of apprenticeship for practitioners (discussed in chapter 3) that was also coupled with magic or often religious aspects, as healing often is even today. By isolating magical (and supposedly Germanic) elements from the classical and others in the texts and pursuing them as isolated elements to literary ends, sight is lost of the medical tradition. It becomes fragmented into many parts, and a view of the whole is distorted.

Appropriating and expanding on Cockayne's ideas, Singer and later Bonser (in even greater detail) separated out classical and "barbaric" elements in medicine as much as possible, seen particularly in Singer's *From Magic to Science* (where, it might be added, Singer's choice of words was remarkably similar to Henry Sigerists's, whose 1923 work on classical and medieval medicine is discussed in the next chapter, but was not mentioned by Singer). For example, Bonser wrote:

> But magic, as will be seen from the following pages, was associated with most branches of medicine, thereby ousting the healing art itself. The assessment of what was of value for healing purposes was therefore entirely different from what it had been in classical Greece and what it is today. Thus one must not necessarily look in a prescription for any physiological effect which the ingredients might have had on a patient. (Bonser, 8)

In chapter 3, several modern scholars are discussed who are studying the physiological effects and bio-chemical properties of medicinal plants and providing scientific explanations as to why many medieval remedies are configured in the way that they are—to ensure that they work and not because they invoke any magical power.

In a summary statement, Bonser's teacher, Singer, said, "The magic and medicine of Early England must be studied as a whole if we wish to learn something of the cultural factors that have gone to make up this remarkable system, or to gain a true picture of the attitude of the inhabitants of this country towards the healing art, before the arrival of that scholastic method and Arabian learning which wrought nearly as great a mental revolution in the thirteenth, as the experimental method and scientific attitude in the seventeenth century" (Singer, *Science*, 136–7). (It should be noted that medical historian John Riddle believes the scholastic approach to medicine actually hurt herbal prescriptions, since they then became part of a complex world of theory divorced from practice.)[18] In actuality, Singer's goal was apparently to see not the whole, but the parts, and to expose each to scathing ridicule. Bonser, like Cockayne and Singer but in more detail, discussed the folkloric, magical, anecdotal, literary, and ostensibly scientific aspects of medieval medicine as evidenced by a welter of details, none of which painted a picture of what actual practice might have been as a whole. One allegedly scientific

introduction to a discussion of skin disease bears quoting in this regard
because it is typical for Bonser: "It becomes obvious from a study of Anglo-
Saxon medicine that, generally speaking, the interior of the body was then
practically unknown, and that its exterior claimed most of the attention of the
leech. The number of recipes for skin diseases is therefore large" (Bonser,
369). The causes of such disease are said to be "neglect of personal hygiene"
based on "abundant evidence," none of which is cited.

Singer's view was that the magical folk practices of the Germanic peoples, which they had brought from the Continent, gave way before the written
word of classical medicine. However, he characterized the magic as barbaric
and preposterous and the classical as decayed Greek science that was mind-
lessly copied. This characterization reinforced the notion of distinct traditions, which tended to fragment the way in which medieval medicine was
viewed. It also created the untenable notion that Latin- and Greek-based texts
like the *Herbarium* were for some reason copied in the scriptoria but never
used in medieval Europe. Of the remedies in the Anglo-Saxon medical texts,
particularly the *Herbarium*, he said:

> It would be an error to regard all the elaborate prescriptions in these writ-
> ings as indicating the actual lines of treatment. For practical reasons many
> of the recipes could not have been prepared. Any leech who claimed that he
> had so prepared them would have been guilty of fraud. *In fact dark age
> medical manuscripts are partly mere literary material and in places hardly
> more than scribal exercises. They are always unintelligently copied* and the
> prescriptions are often mere elaborate displays of learning. Many of the
> remedies that they set forth were completely unintelligible to the leeches of
> the time; others involved preparations altogether beyond their meager tech-
> nical skill [emphasis added]. (Singer, *Science*, 24)

Singer offered scant proof for his claims, and his statements were made with
little appeal to what was in the texts—except for the charms. Bonser built on
this notion.

It appears to have been Singer who introduced the idea that the *Herbarium* was a "mere" translation of a classical text that was for reasons unknown
slavishly copied; he may have derived the notion from Cockayne's estimation of the intellectual capacity of the leeches to learn from the classical
world. At any rate, Singer was careful to isolate the native Anglo-Saxon and
Germanic lore from what was assumed to be the bookish, classical medical
tradition. The argument presented here is that although vestiges of early Germanic lore are somewhat more evident in the *Lacnunga* and *Bald's Leechbook,* the two other Anglo-Saxon medical texts, evidence points to the fact
that by the time these texts were written and the *Herbarium of Pseudo-
Apuleius* was translated into Old English, a composite, distinctly medieval
tradition had been established throughout Europe, and the *Herbarium, Bald's*

Leechbook, and the *Lacnunga* all belonged to it (as discussed in more detail in chapter 3).

The argument made here challenges the neat division of medieval medicine into classical and barbaric, a categorization suggested in Cockayne that was made into law by Singer and continued in Bonser and others. To the contrary, the present work shows that by the early medieval period, practical medicine had fused classical and "barbaric" elements (which included Roman superstition) into one tradition, which is reflected in the *Herbarium* and the other two Anglo-Saxon texts. However, enabled by Cockayne's editions and translations of all the Anglo-Saxon medical texts and following Cockayne's and Singer's suggestions, scholars in search of what can be considered unique to Anglo-Saxon folklore and folk medicine have deemed the supposedly classical *Herbarium* useless to early England and have declared the *Leechbook* and *Lacnunga* to be goldmines of hidden information about the native culture. The thesis of the present work is that to understand the medical practice of Anglo-Saxon England, it must be studied in the context of the Continental tradition to which it clearly belonged. Moreover, the tradition must be seen as a whole to be understood, not broken into hypothetical parts that are allegedly Teutonic, Celtic, classical, and the like. In addition, one basis for the argument is that there is no reliable way to isolate pristine elements characterizing *Ur*-Anglo-Saxon culture as distinct from a general Indo-European one.

The assumption that the *Herbarium* and works like it were not useful medical texts was stated more or less as received knowledge in the two unpublished dissertations mentioned earlier. Frieda Hankins, for example, listed the main sources for knowledge of Anglo-Saxon medicine and magic only as MSS Harley 585 and Royal 12.D.xviii, because the *Lacnunga* and *Bald's Leechbook* are in them, and she characterized the *Herbarium* merely as "an Anglo-Saxon translation from the Greek Apuleius . . . a description of herbs and plants" (Hankins, 2). Singer was nearly alone in thinking the *Herbarium* came from the Greek, and the original is generally accepted to have been in Latin. Likewise, in speaking about Cockayne's translations of the medical texts from Anglo-Saxon England, Barbara Olds claimed that "[o]f all these writings, the most studied and the most useful for an understanding of Anglo-Saxon medicine are the *Lacnunga* and *Leechbook*" (Olds, 2). Of the *Herbarium*, Olds said it was a compilation based on Pliny, written in North Africa at the end of the fifth century. Published works continue the assumed distinction, such as a recent work by Karen Jolly, in which what is called "rational" or "classical" medicine in the *Herbarium* is contrasted unfavorably with what is considered to be useful "native" material in the *Lacnunga* and *Bald's Leechbook*.[19]

Both Olds and Hankins also cited Charles Talbot's *Medicine in Medieval England,* a work that claimed *Bald's Leechbook* and the *Lacnunga* were important because they reflected actual practice. Talbot's work placed the *Herbarium* in the category of classical (sometimes referred to as rational) medicine and the author mentioned it almost as an aside to the two other works. At the same time, however, Talbot acknowledged the known and suspected classical sources that can be found everywhere in *Bald's Leechbook* and also in the *Lacnunga*. Talbot's argument is that when the Romans left England, all that remained for the Saxons to encounter were "the descendants of the serfs who had clustered in villages on the outskirts of the Roman cities. . . . Like all primitive peoples the Saxons had some knowledge of herbs and a rudimentary acquaintance with surgery. But it was more empirical than rational, overlaid with magic and superstition and rooted in folklore. This was to persist long after the introduction of what is called rational medicine."[20]

Talbot postulated that classical, which he called rational, medicine could have come to England with Theodore of Tarsus and could have been taught at his school at Canterbury. Moreover, he devoted considerable space to the medical writing that by then existed on the Continent and could have been available to the Anglo-Saxons through the system of monks and monasteries who were the keepers and transmitters of texts, and were also serving as medical healers. He listed the standard authors of these classical texts, and complimented highly the contents in *Bald's Leechbook* that came from these authors. For example: "The Leech-Book embodies the teaching of Greek writers as transmitted by Latin translations. . . . In short, far from the Leech-Book being a tissue of folk remedies and irrational ideas, it embodies some of the best medical literature available to the West at that time. . . . Indeed even the irrational remedies which appear from time to time in the Leech-book are the same as those used by Galen and Celsus" (Talbot, 18–19).

When evaluating the *Lacnunga*, Talbot echoed Cockayne and Singer in expressing his complete certainty that a society capable of producing the likes of Ælfric and Wulfstan would have had "little place" for such superstition and magic. His conclusion on the work was, "[t]o lay great emphasis, then, on a single extravagant text like the *Lacnunga* is to throw everything out of perspective." This is true; however it is misleading for Talbot, like Singer and Bonser, to find Greek, Roman, Byzantine, Celtic, and Teutonic sources for this work alone, since such sources are typical for early medieval medicine and its combination of the rational, folklore, and magic. (Talbot cited only two sources for his chapter on Anglo-Saxon medicine: the 1904 work by J. F. Payne, *English Medicine in Anglo-Saxon Times*, and Grattan and Singer's *Anglo-Saxon Magic and Medicine*.) The modern fixation with data collection in subdivided and precise compartments fosters such fragmentation, to the point that one may lose sight of the tradition as a whole.[21]

In contrast to the trend established by Cockayne and Singer, and continued by Bonser and others, not everyone sees a neat distinction between classical medicine and magical native Germanic practices. A study by Faye Getz, though concentrating on late medieval medicine in England, stresses the interrelationship of Latin and vernacular medical texts in Anglo-Saxon England and traces what she termed an encyclopedic medical tradition from the ruins of Rome through the early Middle Ages, one which encompassed magic in its early stages. Getz described it as combining medicinal herbs, simple remedies, and charms, and linked it to the medical tradition of the Benedictine monasteries and the texts associated with them (which included all the Anglo-Saxon texts).[22]

Two conferences also pointed up the union of magic and medicine in the medieval period. D. G. Scragg, one of the organizers of the 1987 and 1988 conferences on medieval medicine at Manchester, England, wrote in an introduction to some of the papers published after the conference: "No one in Anglo-Saxon England would have distinguished magic and medicine in the way that we do today, and it was logical therefore that, after the successful conference in Manchester in 1987 on Anglo-Saxon medicine, there should be a follow-up conference to look at magic and at those credited with supernatural healing powers."[23] The eight papers in the two publications cover a wide range of medical subjects, and treatments using herbs are mentioned in many. The conferences are mentioned here to underscore their focus on medicine and magic together.

What emerges from many of the writings reviewed here, beginning with Cockayne, is that modern studies often try to understand past traditions by breaking them into their parts: with medieval medicine split into Greek, Roman, Germanic, magic, folkloric traditions, and so forth. One part of the medieval medical tradition has received a disproportionate amount of attention, beginning again with Singer's appropriations from Cockayne, and that is magic. However, to a great extent, it is clear that the understanding of what is alleged to be magic in Anglo-Saxon (and medieval medicine generally) is based on false assumptions. Cockayne fostered a search for magic; for example in the preface to his volume 1 (1965), he described the medicine of the northern leeches during the "rudest ages" as being a combination of medicinal plants, charms, and incantations (xxvii). He then likened the superstition of the Germanic tribes to superstitious practices of the Roman Church in the "earlier ages of our modern period" (xxviii), practices such as "medicine masses, and blessing of worts out in the field." He quoted Germanic and Scandinavian sources to show the widespread belief in the power of witches, dwarfs, wizards, even by such people as Bede and Theodorus, Archbishop of Canterbury.

Godfrid Storms, however, challenged the idea that magic or, even more specifically, pagan magic, could easily be identified as such in medieval medical texts (in this he echoes Payne, discussed earlier). In *Anglo-Saxon Magic,* Storms discussed magic, its origins, and how magic was used to heal;

hence, the two Anglo-Saxon manuscripts with the most magic, *Bald's Leech-book* and *Lacnunga*, are the center of the study.[24] (The *Herbarium* was not excluded, and a number of its remedies are said to have a magic element.) Storms was early in tying all three Anglo-Saxon medical texts to a pan-European tradition with the goal of finding the *Ur*-Germanic and the *Ur*-Indo-European in them, a quest not unlike Sir James George Frazer's in the *Golden Bough*, which he cited. However, Storms clearly stated how difficult it is to separate the native from the classical sources in any of this material. (Singer, on the other hand, said that certain ancient elements were discernible in the Anglo-Saxon *Lacnunga*, but included no evidence.)

Of particular relevance with regard to Singer and those who followed him in seeking the native in the Old English medical texts is the careful approach Storms took in his chapter 5, where he attempted to distinguish Anglo-Saxon, classical, and Christian elements in the magico-medical texts. He said that the Anglo-Saxons had no general denomination for magic, nor did the Romans, and found that Anglo-Saxon expressions mainly referred to the way in which the magic actions were performed, rather than to magic in general. He said that they used abstract terms made with *-craeft* to describe magical practices. In addition, Storms thought that it was relatively easy to recognize and distinguish Christian from pagan elements, but much more difficult to separate pagan Germanic elements from pagan classical elements.

Singer identified four unique elements that he believed distinguished pagan Teutonic ideas about the cause of disease: (1) flying venoms, (2) the evil nines, (3) worm as the cause of disease, and (4) the doctrine of elf-shot (Singer, *Magic*, 52–62). With regard to the first three, which are interrelated as Singer explained it, the god of health and good luck, Woden, smashed the serpent or worm, the symbol of death, into nine pieces, and these pieces produced nine venoms that fly through the air and cause disease. He cited references to these three doctrines particularly in the *Lacnunga*. Singer described in some detail how dwarfs and elves were blamed for disease in the pages cited. However Storms concluded that with the exception of the last, elf-shot, "we can hardly speak of distinguishing characteristics because the same elements occur in classical magic as well, as was admitted by Singer" (Storms, 118). Whereas Singer thought the Anglo-Saxons brought these four elements of magic with them from their Continental homes to England, Storms found them to be part of a common pool of Indo-European information—not characteristically Anglo-Saxon—saying: "If we find a well-developed vernacular formula whose contents do not point to a foreign source, we can be sure that it is a true Germanic charm." In fact, Storms thought that even if the existence of an Anglo-Saxon tradition could be established, it need not differ from that of Italy and Greece, and to back this up said, "If some charm or practice is recorded by Marcellus or Alexander of Tralles, it may still be of Teutonic origin, because they both spent part of their life among Teutonic tribes, and they were influenced by Teutonic superstition" (Storms, 121).

The modern practice of isolating the *Old English Herbarium* from the other Anglo-Saxon medical texts because it is thought to be "classical" has tended to diminish the importance of the *Herbarium* to its time and as a part of the medical tradition of Anglo-Saxon England. Cockayne's prefaces to the *Leechdoms* laid the foundations for this isolation, which is echoed in later scholars studying the Anglo-Saxon medical texts. A. J. Minnis spoke about contextualization and medieval literary texts, and his thoughts clearly apply here. In his *Medieval Theory of Authorship*, Minnis wrote, "Cultural change is one thing: cultural imperialism is something else. One can only hope that the greater awareness of medieval literary theory and criticism will help us go back to the texts and their contexts with the desire to listen and learn, not to shout down and dominate."[25]

This study has Minnis's admonition in mind in looking at the legacy of Cockayne's *Leechdoms, Wortcunning, and Starcraft of Early England* and in the placement of the *Old English Herbarium* in the pantheon of Anglo-Saxon medical texts. Looking at this work only as a rational, classical work has tended wrongly to isolate it from the supposedly more native *Lacnunga* and *Bald's Leechbook*. In the following chapter, the *Herbarium of Pseudo-Apuleius* is studied as part of an early European medical tradition to which it and the Old English version belong, and it becomes clear that the *Old English Herbarium* must be put back on the shelf beside the *Lacnunga* and the *Leechbook* as texts that were valuable for understanding their time. (In all fairness, the Latin medical manuscripts from the same period must be included too.) All belonged to the same basic tradition, just with a different mix of sources. The texts in Anglo-Saxon England were found throughout the monastery libraries of Europe, with the same evidence for their having been used. J. D. A. Ogilvy characterized the *Herbarium of Pseudo-Apuleius* as "[a]pparently the standard medical text of the later Anglo-Saxons. . . . It is really a complex of Dioscorides, Pseudo-Apuleius, Pseudo-Musa (*De Herba Bettonica, De Taxone*) and Sectus Placitus Papyriensis *De Med. ex Animalibus.*"[26] By the time it was translated into Old English, the *Herbarium* complex in England also included the additions and revisions of those who had copied, translated, and used it over the years.

Cockayne's Translations as Transformations

Cockayne's prefaces to the *Leechdoms* and his translation style set the stage for reading the Anglo-Saxon medical texts as literary curiosities, nothing more. Cockayne viewed the Anglo-Saxons as cultural children, lacking the refinements and medical skill of the classical world, and as a result his "translations" were actually transformations of the Anglo-Saxon medical texts. For the *Old English Herbarium*, Cockayne transformed it into what might be called Cockayne's *Herbarium*, whose legacy continues today.

That such transformations are not unusual is the message in Lawrence Venuti's book, *The Scandals of Translation*. The work illustrates how a translation can intentionally influence the way a different culture will receive the original, and the argument presented is that translations reflect the translator's perception/reception not only of the work itself, but of the culture from which the work comes.[27] (Venuti's primary interest was literary translations and the problems in translating—or failures to translate—the literature of marginalized cultures. In many ways, Cockayne saw Anglo-Saxon culture as marginal, in our words, as a third-world country.) Venuti argued that the choice of words, the omissions, the paraphrases, the adaptations involved in translating any text, but particularly literature, from one language to another constitute a reworking of the original text, no matter how "literal" the translation is intended to be. He wrote:

> Translation wields enormous power in constructing representations of foreign cultures. Foreign literatures tend to be dehistoricized by the selection of texts for translation, removed from the foreign literary traditions where they draw their significance. . . . Translation patterns that come to be fairly established fix stereotypes for foreign cultures, excluding values, debates, and conflicts that don't appear to serve domestic agendas. (Venuti, *Scandals*, 67)

Although Venuti was primarily concerned with modern literature and the effect of translations on how foreign texts are received in dominant cultures, his ideas are very much applicable to Cockayne's treatment of Anglo-Saxon works. Cockayne's translations should not be seen simply as translations but as appropriations of "foreign" (read historical) texts by a dominant culture. They are creations of a nineteenth-century antiquarian whose historical prejudices and stereotypes are obvious.

Two recent works dealing specifically with the influence of nineteenth-century scholarship on Anglo-Saxon studies help explain why Cockayne transformed the medical texts with which he worked (albeit unintentionally), and why his ideas and Singer's have gained such ready acceptance. In *The Search for Anglo-Saxon Paganism*, E. G. Stanley discussed a quest in Anglo-Saxon studies to find the pagan Germanic, a discussion that pertains to the foregoing review of what has occurred in studies of the medieval medical texts. Stanley's thesis is that "[f]or a long time Old English literature was much read in the hope of discovering in it a lost world of pre-Christian antiquity, for the reconstruction of which the Old English writings themselves do not provide sufficient fragments."[28] Stanley pointed out that modern followers of Jacob Grimm have tried to exclude all Christian elements

from interpretations and sources of Anglo-Saxon *literary* works in an effort
to remove this "veneer" from the pagan underpinnings (Stanley, 1).

Stanley's explanation of how Grimm and his followers used mythologi-
cal etymology to back up their literary conclusions sheds much light on comments often made about such works as the *Lacnunga* (Cockayne used the
same kind of word tracing):

> The use of the poetic vocabulary of the Anglo-Saxons to illustrate the con-
> tinuity of pagan concepts even after the introduction of Christianity is a fea-
> ture of much of Jacob Grimm's philological work; and following his
> example it became a standard feature of Anglo-Saxon scholarship. For
> example, Grimm asserts that phrases like *hilde woma* are redolent of pagan-
> ism because *woma* is etymologically connected with *Omi*, one of the Norse
> names of Odin, and means "a noise" like that of an approaching God. The
> element of noise aroused a feeling of awe and the sense of a god's immedi-
> ate presence; as Woden was also called Woma, and Oðon also Omi and
> Yggr, so the expressions *woma, sweg, broga*, and *egesa* are used by the
> Anglo-Saxon poets almost synonymously for spirits and divine manifesta-
> tions (from *Deutsche Mythologie* 1844). (Stanley, 17)

Cockayne's fanciful etymologies in *Spoon and Sparrow*, derivations that are
very much like Grimm's in intent, are discussed in chapter 1. In fact, Stanley
specifically mentioned Cockayne and the medical text *Lacnunga* in this connection: "Thunor is never mentioned in the Anglo-Saxon charms, but Cockayne supplied that want by emendation and was followed, though with a
different interpretation, by Bosworth under *fyrgen* in his *Dictionary*" (Stanley, 90).

Like Stanley, Allen J. Frantzen in his provocative *Desire for Origins: New
Language, Old English, and Teaching the Tradition* examined in detail the fundamental role of nineteenth-century scholarship to modern trends in Anglo-
Saxon studies. Though Frantzen's purpose in writing the book was to examine
critically what these foundations have meant to modern scholarship, he
brought out certain points about the seminal years of Anglo-Saxon studies in
Germany and England in the nineteenth century whose repercussions can be
traced to modern critical attitudes toward the three Anglo-Saxon medical texts.
These attitudes have led to regarding the *Herbarium* as (merely) a translation
from the Latin, *Bald's Leechbook* as a composite with some "native" elements,
and the *Lacnunga* as of relatively pure, native Germanic derivation. Frantzen's
underlying thesis is that we create the origins we seek. Frantzen called for a
consideration of memory and oral tradition (neither of them written), and the
fact that Latin and Old English were used by the same people at the same time
in interpreting written texts. About translations, he said, "We know that the textual relations of Anglo-Saxon literary culture were more complex than the simple translation model ("from" Latin "to" Anglo-Saxon) allows."[29]

   This issue of creation versus translation, which reaches into hermeneutics, goes far beyond the scope of this study, as do the larger issues of translation theory. However translation per se merits brief discussion, even though
the primary texts of concern are Cockayne's translations of scientific (nonlit-
erary) works, where accuracy and impartiality rather than literary interpretation and the issue of authorial intent are the major concern. Indeed, few
works on translation theory deal with the topic of translations of scientific
works, favoring literary translations entirely because of the problems they
create with literary interpretation. (An especially provocative discussion of
Venuti's targets the largely unacknowledged problems associated with studying literature in translation, which is so prevalent in schools and universities.
In *Scandals of Translation*, Venuti asserted that discussion is seldom raised
about the problems associated with studying a translation, which is an inter-
pretation or a new work based on the original. See especially his chapter 5,
"The Pedagogy of Literature.")
   The issue of faithful translation versus paraphrase is, of course, not new.
In *Rhetoric, Hermeneutics, and Translation in the Middle Ages,* Rita
Copeland wrote:

> [During the Roman Empire] Rhetoric sought to establish itself as the mas-
> ter discipline, the province of textual or oratorical production, relegating to
> grammar that of language use and glossing and interpretation of the poets.
> Cicero originated the "non verbum pro verbo" concept in *De optimo genere
> oratorum* 5.14–15. Jerome and others passed it on. To translate as an orator
> in the profession of rhetoric, means one can exercise the productive power
> of rhetoric—not just as a grammarian who only should translate word for
> word because their duty is to "practice within the restricted competence of
> the textual critic whose duty is to gloss word for word."[30]

Copeland restricted her study to academic critical discourse in Latin and vernacular traditions, that is, to the academic study and reception of ancient *auc-
tores*. As she observed: "My arguments do not necessarily extend to the
emergence of popular translation in genres such as the *lai* or the metrical
romance from one vernacular language to another, nor to hagiographical or
devotional writings, nor to translation of scientific or technical works"
(Copeland, 5). But in her discussion of translation as belonging either to
rhetoric (*inventio*, creation/paraphrase) or to grammar (*ennaratio*, literal/word-
for-word), Copeland was exploring much the same territory as Venuti, simply
in a different age. And, although describing medieval translation strategies,
Copeland could have been talking about Cockayne's translation of the Anglo-
Saxon medical texts here: "A chief maneuver of academic hermeneutics is to
displace the very text that it proposes to serve" (Copeland, 3). Cockayne's style
of translating transformed the Anglo-Saxon text from a medical reference written in a reasonably plain style into fanciful literary arcana.

Presenting the same argument for the Anglo-Saxon age, Janet Bately showed in her 1980 lecture "The Literary Prose of King Alfred's Reign: Translation or Transformation?" that already in the age of King Alfred (ninth-century England) when the *Herbarium* was almost certainly in England and may well have been a candidate for translation, the issue of literal translation versus paraphrase versus adaptation into *Englisc* was certainly a concern, though again, primarily for literary or philosophical works, not expressly for medicine and science.[31] In fact, in using Alfred's famous description of his translation technique—*hwilum worde be worde, hwilum andgit of angiete*—in the preface to Alfred's translation of Gregory's *Pastoral Care*, Bately introduced a discussion of whether the literary prose of Alfred's reign was actually translation or instead a transformation. Her conclusion was that "[j]ust as Alfred's wood-gatherer took it [wood] from more than one source and transformed it into a fair dwelling for the refreshment of the body, so the king himself and at least one other translator of his reign shaped their source material for the refreshment of the mind, and discarding literal translation transformed the Latin into what may be called independent English prose" (Bately, 21). By interpreting difficult Latin passages for the reader as they "translated" passages into English, the translators of Alfred's time tended to be actually transformers, Bately found.

The transformations have continued. For example, Josephine Helm Bloomfield suggested that Frederick Klaeber's venerated edition of *Beowulf* (1922) strongly reflects values in Prussian Germany at the turn of the twentieth century, a situation analogous to what Cockayne did with the medieval medical texts. Klaeber favored "kind" and "kindness" in notes, articles, and glosses when the words used referred to Queen Wealhtheow, Bloomfield argued, but elsewhere, in masculine contexts, those same words were given such meanings as "lordly," "glorious," and "fitting." Klaeber did not alter the character of Wealhtheow by conscious intent, Bloomfield suggested, but explained that he (like Cockayne) was shaped by his own culture and it necessarily affected his scholarship. Bloomfield wrote, "Even a scholar so great as he [Klaeber] might not have been able to escape or override the influences of his own culture in such areas as gender and gender roles (or indeed in such areas as family relationships and political authority)."[32]

Transformation is an apt term for Cockayne's translations of literary and technical texts; and the argument presented here is that in the case of the Anglo-Saxon medical texts, the transformations have negatively influenced the reception of these works in the modern world. Yet although outrageously convoluted at times, Cockayne's translations were in tune with literary trends in England at the time, trends toward escapism into earlier eras, especially the Middle Ages, as seen in the works of, for example, Sir Walter Scott, John Keats, Samuel Taylor Coleridge, Robert Browning, Dante Gabriel Rossetti (Rossetti and his brother were pupils at King's College School at about the time Cockayne may have first taught there, 1837–41), William Morris, and Alfred Lord Tennyson. Unfortunately, although he never talked about translation theory per se, Cockayne consciously chose a style that was controversial, was never particularly praised, and quickly went out of vogue, one whose intent was to recall a bygone era, such as Anglo-Saxon England, by its use of antiquated words and turns of phrase.

In the mid-1860s, the time when Cockayne was translating the Anglo-Saxon medical texts, a literary dispute about the best way to translate ancient works occurred. In chapter 3 in a volume on the history of translation, Lawrence Venuti termed it the war between proponents of "fluent translation" (championed by Matthew Arnold) and "foreignizing translations" (embraced by F. W. Newman, the Pre-Raphaelites, and William Morris),[33] but the essential question was whether literalism or poetry should prevail in a translation, in this case, of Homer. In this book, Venuti was studying how translation can be seen as a locus of difference, finding that the Victorian elite used fluent translation to strengthen upper-class values. Fluent translation erases the differences; foreignizing emphasizes them. It is clear that Arnold and Newman differed on the audience for noble poetry such as Homer, with Arnold holding scholars as the audience and arbiter of taste, Newman aiming at average readers, feeling this was also Homer's audience.

According to Venuti, Newman ([1805–97] brother of the Cardinal) challenged the main line of English-language translation in his 1856 translation of Homer's *Iliad*, because he "adopted a discourse that signified historical remoteness—archaism. He argues against a modern style for ancient works in translation. He even argues for using 'Saxo-Norman' for Homer, because his [Homer's] style is nearer the old English ballad [style] than the polished verse of Pope" (Venuti, *History*, 122–23). Venuti characterized Newman's translations as "rich stew drawn from various literary discourses" (Venuti, *History*, 124), and, in fact, Newman published a glossary with his translation to define the archaic terms he used. Newman considered his translation to be a faithful imitation of Homer's style and diction, which he said ranged from the popular to the noble, from the archaic to modern, thus to Newman's mind justifying his use of archaic terms and ballad meter; in other words, creating a rather popular poem, because the original was popular (and noble) and came from an heroic age.

> [Homer's] beauty, when it is at its height, is wild beauty: it smells of the mountain and of the sea. If he be compared to a noble animal, it is not to such a spruce rubbed-down Newmarket racer as our smooth translators would pretend, but to a wild horse of the Don Cossacks; and if I, instead of this, present to the reader nothing but a Dandie Dinmont's pony, this, as a first approximation, is a valuable step towards the true solution. . . . I regard it as a question about to open hereafter, whether a translator of Homer ought not to adopt the old disyllabic landis, houndis, hartis, etc., instead of

our modern unmelodious lands, hounds, harts; whether the ye or y before
the past participle may not be restored; the want of which confounds that
participle with the past tense. Even the final en of the plural of verbs (we
dancen, they singen, etc.) still subsists in Lancashire.[34]

Matthew Arnold (1822–88), the Oxford professor of poetry and literary
critic, thought Newman's was a very bad translation—so bad that he roundly
criticized it in a lecture series published as *On Translating Homer* in 1861.
The pejorative term "to Newmanize" originated in this lecture; Arnold
"coined a satiric neologism for Newman's translation discourse—to "Newmanize"—and for the next twenty-five years this word was part of the lexicon of critical terms in the literary periodicals" (Venuti, *History*, 140).
Leading literary magazines kept the subject alive, and it is reasonable to
assume that Cockayne was aware of the controversy though he nowhere
addressed translation style. Arnold spoke up for poetry, assailing Newman's
style and forced diction, claiming that in his effort to be true to the original,
Newman created something that was based on wrong principles and, most
importantly of all, was displeasing to the modern reader of English.

> Mr. Newman says [in his introduction to his translation of the *Iliad*] that
> "the entire dialect of Homer being essentially archaic, that of a translator
> ought to be as much Saxo-Norman as possible, and owe as little as possible
> to the elements thrown into our language by classical learning." Mr. New-
> man is unfortunate in the observance of his own theory; for I continually
> find in his translation words of Latin origin, which seem to me quite alien to
> the simplicity of Homer—"responsive," for instance, which is a favourite
> word of Mr Newman, to represent the Homeric ἀμειβόμενος: "Great Hec-
> tor of the motely helm thus spake to her responsive./But thus responsively
> to him spake godlike Alexander."[35]

Also involved in the dispute, largely by choosing Newman's style of
translation, was William Morris (1834–96). Among the endeavors for which
he is famous are decidedly *not* his translations of ancient and medieval works
(published roughly between 1860 and 1895), which used this archaic style.
In a recent book on Morris by Paul Thompson, all of these translations merit
only about two paragraphs of commentary.

> Morris's verse translations, like his prose versions of the sagas, miss the
> essential qualities for success, clarity, and readability. They are accurate
> translations, but so carefully kept to the original lines and order of phrases
> that they are difficult to read. For the *Aeneid* and the *Odyssey* Morris relied
> on his own Greek and Latin, but for *Beowulf* he had the help of a Cam-
> bridge scholar, A. J. Wyatt. It is perhaps the worst thing he ever wrote, quite
> incomprehensible without a glossary.[36]

Echoing this evaluation, Venuti said that *Longman's Magazine* called Morris's translations "Wardour-Street Early English," a kind of sham antique. The periodical questioned the authenticity of his archaism and linked it to nonstandard English and marginal literary forms: "Poems in which guests go bedward to beds that are arrayed right meet, poems in which thrall-folk seek to the feast-hall a-winter, do not belong to any literary centre. They are provincial, they are utterly without distinction, they are unspeakably absurd" (Venuti, *History*, 14, quoting *Longman's Magazine* 12 (Oct) 1888: 585–94).

Cockayne died before Morris's translations of Homer, Virgil, and *Beowulf* appeared; however, he might have known Morris and Eirikr Magnusson's 1869 translation of the *Volsunga Saga*, the first into English, or some of Morris's earlier works either translated from or based on the Nordic sagas. In *Sigurd the Volsung* (1876), Morris created an epic that "was based on medieval forms, but combined with a wholly new freedom. Morris wrote it in rhymed couplets, binding the long lines with frequent alliteration" (Thompson, 198). Thompson considered this " a great poem, an epic of truly heroic stature. Today it is acknowledged, but little read. . . . It is set in the world of the sagas, but its values are those of Morris, not the Norsemen" (Thompson, 202). The latter part of this estimation applies equally to Cockayne's *Leechdoms.* Though Morris cannot be really linked to Cockayne in any conclusive way, Cockayne translated in a style very much like that of Morris. The style was embraced by some of his contemporaries, writers and scholars who were interested in ancient and medieval languages and who sought to transmit some of the flavor of remote ages to the present (many, such as Morris and Newman, for political reasons). Earlier, the historian Sharon Turner advocated and used an archaic style in translating Anglo-Saxon poems (*Beowulf* among them), most of which are in volume 3 of his *History of the Anglo-Saxons*. He said that his translations were "literally faithful, in order that the style, as well as the sense, of the Anglo-Saxon writer might be perceived" (Turner, 1:vi). Cockayne clearly belonged to this well-established tradition of archaizing translation, which went out of vogue even as he was using it. Anyone who uses the Loeb Library editions of the Latin and Greek authors is well-acquainted with archaizing translations.

However, one contemporary review of Cockayne's *Leechdoms*, the only one identified for this work to date, was favorable to its translation style. In what amounts to a fourteen-page essay on ancient and medieval medicine and magic, much of its information gleaned from Cockayne's prefaces without acknowledgment, an unnamed reviewer in the *Dublin University Magazine* for May 1867 wrote:

> The translation fully possesses the compactness and rough strength of the original. Any reader of philological taste will scarcely arise from the persual

of the volumes without a deeper liking for unadulterated English than he
entertained before, so well does it combine clearness, compactness, and
vigour, and fitness.[37]

In dealing with the subject matter of Cockayne's three volumes, however, the
reviewer presaged the interest and biases following decades would bestow on
them: fascination with the magical elements and belief that the alleged medicinal properties of plants was "mystical." Sweet's unfavorable review of
Cockayne's *Juliana* (the only other identified review of Cockayne's work
published in his lifetime) is cited in the previous chapter, with its estimation
that his style makes the Anglo-Saxon work sound ridiculous.

Cockayne's translations of *Hali Meidenhad* and *St. Margaret* (both from
1866) exemplify the archaizing style of translation, for better or worse. Perhaps such a style can be justified for this type of literature, inspirational religious texts from the early Middle Ages. Perhaps Cockayne felt, like Newman
and Morris, that the following would convey a sense of a time far-removed:

> Þus, woman, if þou hast a husband to þy mind and enjoyment, also, of
> worldly weal, must needs happen to þe. And what if it happen, as þe wont
> is, þat þou have neiþer þy will wið him, nor weal eiþer, and must groan
> wiðout goods wiðin waste walls, and in want of bread must breed þy row of
> bairns; and still furþer, viro quem summo odio habes, succumbere, who,
> þough þou hadst all weald, will turn it to sorrow. . . . [38]

From the *Herbarium*:

3. For stirring of the inwards, take this same wort, work it to a salve; lay it
to the sore of the inwards. It also is well beneficial for heartache.
4. For sore of the milt (*spleen*), take juice of this same wort one cup, and
five spoonsful of vinegar; give (this) to drink for nine days; thou wilt wonder at the benefit. Take also the root of the same wort, and hang it about the
mans swere (*neck*), so that it may hang in front against the milt (*spleen*);
soon he will be healed. And whatsoever man swallows the juice of this
wort, with wondrous quickness he will perceive relief of the inwards. This
wort a man may collect at any period. (Cockayne 1965, 1:113; entry XVIII
for cyclamen)

All of Cockayne's translations, including the *Leechdoms*, read this way, and
today the Early English Text Society has replaced his *Hali Meidenhad*,
Juliana, and *St. Marherete*. The fact that they have been replaced does not
mean that his translations were not accurate, but that the style makes them
needlessly difficult to read and understand.

It is unfortunate that Cockayne chose this dense and difficult style for
the medical texts, because scientific texts demand clarity above all, and the
translations in his three-volume *Leechdoms* are, for the most part, so incom-
prehensible to the modern reader that they serve no useful purpose other than
to illustrate examples of medieval superstition. The Old English medical

texts are just now beginning to be taken seriously as the basis for objective studies of medieval medicine and its practice, instead of being used primarily as sources for scholars seeking superstitions and charms. When they have been used at all, Cockayne's translations have primarily been part of literary and, not medical studies, and their content has generally not been used in healing or to understand medieval medical practice or the herbal medical tradition. It might be noted that Singer felt it necessary to provide a new translation of the *Lacnunga* for his *Anglo-Saxon Magic and Medicine* for reasons of style and accuracy.

Already in *Hali Meidenhad*, as seen in the short passage above, Cockayne chose to translate some passages from Anglo-Saxon not into modern English but into Latin, a practice he also followed in the *Leechdoms*. His rationale was this: "Þis treatise on þe high state of virginity contains so many coarse and repulsive passages, þat it was laid out for printing wiþout a modernized version; . . . þe most objectionable portions have been Latinized" (Cockayne *Meidenhad*, v). In some of the texts, gynecological conditions were also too coarse and repulsive, because the Victorian clergyman often ran Latin into his modern English translation, leaving a reader who cannot read the original Anglo-Saxon totally perplexed about what is happening. For example, when translating uses for the plant "conyza," he wrote: "2. This wort conyza, sodden in water, and mulieri sedenti supposita matricem purgat. 3. Si parere mulier nequit, succum huius herbae cum lana ad naturam eius applices, cito partum perficiet" (Cockayne 1965, 1:267). And even when he did translate the entire passage into modern English, the meaning is not always clear: for the sprenge plant (*Euphorbia lathyris*), Cockayne wrote: "For sore of the inwards, take a shrub of this wort tithymallus, pound it in wine, so that of the wine there be two draughts, add then thereto two spoons of the ooze of the wort, let him then drink this fasting; he will be healed" (Cockayne 1965, 1:225). And for yarrow, (*Achillea millefolium*), Cockayne supplied, "In case that any man with difficulty can pass water, take ooze of this same wort with vinegar, give it him to drink; wondrously it healeth" (Cockayne, 1965, 1:195). Although being faithful to the Old English original, Cockayne was not being friendly to the reader of modern English. Literary specialists may have no trouble with such turns of phrase. The *Herbarium,* however, was not intended for this readership, to which it is now largely confined because of Cockayne's translation.

All the works envisioned for the Rolls Series were to round out a history of England from the earliest times, and Cockayne's intent in rescuing the medical/scientific texts from museum storage was to demonstrate practices current during the infancy of the British nation. The prefaces Cockayne wrote for his volumes of the series set the tone for how these texts ought to be received, and in the case of the medical works, he compared them most unfavorably with classical Greek texts and practices, since he believed the Anglo-Saxons incapable of mastering classical medicine. But in suggesting that *Bald's Leechbook* and the *Lacnunga* abounded in charms and magic that were barbaric (hence possibly purely Germanic) and assigning the *Old English Herbarium* to the classical Greek tradition, Cockayne set up an artificial division between the texts that did not exist when they were used, a division he made little of because he was not particularly interested in either the medical or magical content of the texts. Later scholars of Anglo-Saxon language and culture were very interested in the magic and folkloric aspects and made much of them, to the exclusion of the *Old English Herbarium.*

In contrast, on the European continent the *Herbarium of Pseudo-Apuleius,* is regarded as one of several important Latin medical texts that circulated widely in Europe throughout the Middle Ages and into the Renaissance. There, its being translated into Anglo-Saxon is considered to be only part of the long life of this Latin work. In Anglo-Saxon studies, however, the Old English work is regarded (or more often dismissed) as a mere translation of a classical Latin work, hence not particularly valuable to the people who copied it. In reality, the *Herbarium of Pseudo-Apuleius* (thus also the *Old English Herbarium*) is not a purely classical work, but is part of a distinct medical textual tradition that evolved during the early Middle Ages, a tradition to which *Bald's Leechbook* and the *Lacnunga* also belong. The following chapter discusses that tradition and the practices that went with it. They were similar in England and in southern Europe because the medicinal plants and other needed ingredients for remedies could have been grown or obtained everywhere, south to north. An appeal to modern herbology, which has its roots in these same traditions, helps in understanding how the *Herbarium* and other texts might have been used in many geographical locations through many centuries.

Notes

1. See for example Brian Inglis, *A History of Medicine* (Cleveland: World, 1965), hereafter cited in text as Inglis; Lois N. Magner, *A History of Medicine* (New York: Marcel Dekker, 1992), and *Merck's 1899 Manual of the Materia Medica: A Ready Reference Pocket Book for the Practicing Physician* (New York: Merck, 1899).
2. For a riveting account of the history of anesthesia in the West, including a firsthand account of a patient who underwent surgery without it, see E. M. Papper, *Romance, Poetry, and Surgical Sleep: Literature Influences Medicine* (Westport, CT: Greenwood Press, 1995). See also Victor Robinson, *Victory Over Pain: A History of Anesthesia* (New York: Henry Schuman, 1946), which includes classical and medieval attempts at anesthesia, and Thomas E. Keys, *The History of Surgical Anesthesia* (1945; New York: Dover, 1963).
3. See William H. McNeill, *Plagues and Peoples* (New York: Doubleday, 1976), especially chapter 6, "The Ecological Impact of Medical Science and Organi-

zation since 1700," and Alfred W. Crosby, Jr., *The Columbian Exchange: Biological and Cultural Consequences of 1492* (Westport, CT: Greenwood, 1972) for a discussion of nutrition.

4. Erwin H. Ackerknecht, M.D., *A Short History of Medicine* (New York: The Ronald Press, 1955), 195, hereafter cited in text as Ackerknecht.

5. Sabine Baring-Gould, *Early Reminiscences: 1834–1864* (New York: E. P. Dutton, n.d. [1922]), 112–3. The book is a goldmine of information on the minutiae of life during the mid-nineteenth century in England and France. In addition, W. M. Thackeray's *Pendennis* of 1850 describes the life of a contemporary apothecary by that name.

6. Peter Bartrip, "Secret Remedies, Medical Ethics, and the Finances of the British Medical Journal," in Robert Baker, ed., *The Codification of Medical Morality: Historical and Philosophical Studies of the Formalization of Western Medical Morality in the Eighteenth and Nineteenth Centuries*, vol. 2 (Dordrecht: Kluwer Academic, 1995), 191–2; hereafter cited in text as Bartrip.

7. Amanda McQuade Crawford, "Western Herbal History," (Albuquerque: The National College of Phytotherapy, 1996), 20.

8. S. G. B. Stubbs and E. W. Bligh, *Sixty Centuries of Health and Physick*, in their chapter on the early Middle Ages titled "A Thousand Years of Darkness" (London: Sampson, Low, Marsten, 1931), 86.

9. Herbert Maxwell, "Odd Volumes—I," *Blackwood's Edinburgh Magazine* 163 (May 1898): 652–70; hereafter cited in text as Maxwell.

10. We have some precise ideas about surgery in Roman Gaul, but we know absolutely nothing about it for the Celts in the British Isles, and nothing about Irish pharmacopoeia, and generally relatively little about Continental Celtic pharmacopoeia during the classical period outside some references to plants, of which the best known, thanks to Pliny the Elder, is mistletoe. Christian-J. Guyonvarc'h, *Magie, médecine et divination chez les Celtes* (Paris: Payot, 1997), 224.

11. Joseph Frank Payne, *The Fitz-Patrick Lectures for 1903: English Medicine in the Anglo-Saxon Times* (London: Clarendon Press, 1904), 4; hereafter cited in text as Payne.

12. See for example Charles Singer, *From Magic to Science: Essays on the Scientific Twilight* (1928; New York: Dover, 1958); hereafter cited in text as Singer, *Science*, and his "The Herbal in Antiquity," *The Journal of Hellenic Studies* 47 (1927): 1–52.

13. J. H. G. Grattan and Charles Singer, *Anglo-Saxon Magic and Medicine* (London: Oxford University Press, 1952), 94; hereafter cited in text as Singer, *Magic*. Grattan was mainly responsible for the translation of the *Lacnunga* that appears here and for philological work with the Old English texts, as Singer explained in his introduction to this work. That Singer was responsible for the broad theories on medieval medicine is evident from his new preface to Cockayne's *Leechdoms*.

14. Wilifrid Bonser, *The Medical Background of Anglo-Saxon England: A Study in History, Psychology, and Folklore* (London: The Wellcome Historical Medical Library, 1963), 6.

15. Loren MacKinney, *Early Medieval Medicine* (Baltimore: The Johns Hopkins Press, 1937), 57–8; hereafter cited in text as MacKinney.

16. Stanley Rubin, *Medieval English Medicine* (New York: Barnes and Noble, 1974), 14; hereafter cited in text as Rubin.

17. Barbara M. Olds, "The Anglo-Saxon Leechbook III: A Critical Edition and Translation," (Ph.D. diss., University of Denver, 1984); hereafter cited in text as Olds. Freda Richards Hankins, "*Bald's Leechbook* Reconsidered," (Ph.D. diss., University of North Carolina at Chapel Hill, 1991); hereafter cited in text as Hankins.

18. See John Riddle, *Contraception and Abortion from the Ancient World to the Renaissance* (Cambridge, MA: Harvard University Press, 1992).

19. Karen Louise Jolly, *Popular Religion in Late Saxon England: Elf Charms in Context* (Chapel Hill: University of North Carolina Press, 1996), see especially 105. Although Jolly talked here about a composite and partly unwritten medical tradition, for some reason she excluded the *Herbarium* and works like it entirely from the realm of medicine as it was practiced in Anglo-Saxon England.

20. C. H. Talbot, *Medicine in Medieval England* (London: Oldbourne, 1967), 9–10; hereafter cited in text as Talbot.

21. For a discussion of the texts that were available to Anglo-Saxon healers, see for example M. L. Cameron, "The Sources of Medical Knowledge in Anglo-Saxon England," *Anglo-Saxon England* 11 (1983): 135–55

22. Faye Getz, *Medicine in the English Middle Ages* (Princeton: Princeton University Press, 1998). See in particular her chapter 3, "Medieval English Medical Texts." What Getz called the encyclopedic tradition appears to be the same that Jerry Stannard and others called *Rezeptliteratur*, a genre discussed in detail in chapter 3. Getz did not reference Stannard or the standard writers on *Rezeptliteratur*, although she did cite Bonser, who mentioned the genre in several places.

23. D. G. Scragg, *Superstition and Popular Medicine in Anglo-Saxon England* (Manchester: University of Manchester, 1989), 7. A companion volume is Marilyn Deegan and D. G. Scragg, eds., *Medicine in Early Medieval England* (Manchester: University of Manchester, 1989).

24. G. Storms, *Anglo-Saxon Magic* (1948; The Hague: Martinus Nijhoff, 1974); hereafter cited in text as Storms.

25. A. J. Minnis, *Medieval Theory of Authorship*, 2nd ed., (Philadelphia: University of Pennsylvania Press, 1984), xvii–xviii.

26. J. D. A. Ogilvy, *Books Known to the English, 597–1066* (Cambridge, MA: Medieval Academy of America, 1967), 75.

27. Lawrence Venuti, *The Scandals of Translation: Towards an Ethics of Difference* (London: Routledge, 1998); hereafter cited in text as Venuti, *Scandals*. See also Eugene A. Nida and William D. Reyburn, *Meaning Across Cultures* (Maryknoll, NY: Orbis Books, 1981) for supporting arguments that translators evaluate what they are translating in terms of the biases of their own culture, and this bias is necessarily reflected in the translation.

28. E. G. Stanley, *The Search for Anglo-Saxon Paganism* (Cambridge: D. S. Brewer, 1975), viii; hereafter cited in text as Stanley. The contents was originally published as articles in *Notes and Queries* (1964–65).

29. Allen J. Frantzen, *Desire for Origins: New Language, Old English, and Teaching the Tradition* (New Brunswick and London: Rutgers University Press, 1990), 87.

30. Rita Copeland, *Rhetoric, Hermeneutics, and Translation in the Middle Ages: Academic Traditions and Vernacular Texts* (Cambridge: Cambridge University Press, 1991), 2; hereafter cited in text as Copeland.

31. Janet Bately, "The Literary Prose of King Alfred's Reign: Translation or Transformation?" (Inaugural Lecture in the Chair of English Language and Medieval Literature delivered at University of London King's College on 4 March 1980); hereafter cited in text as Bately.

32. Josephine Helm Bloomfield, "Diminished by Kindness: Frederick Klaeber's Rewriting of Wealhtheow," *Journal of English and Germanic Philology* 93 (April 1994): 186. See also Bloomfield's "The Canonization of Editorial Sensibility in Beowulf: A Philological and Historical Reassessment of Klaeber's Edition," (Ph.D. diss., University of California at Davis, 1991) for a fuller discussion of Klaeber's bias in the editing of *Beowulf.*

33. Lawrence Venuti, *The Translator's Invisibility: A History of Translation* (London: Routledge, 1995); hereafter cited in text at Venuti, *History.*

34. F. W. Newman, "Homeric Translation in Theory and Practice," in Matthew Arnold, *On Translating Homer: With F. W. Newman's 'Homeric Translation' and Arnold's 'Last Words'* (London: George Routledge and Sons, n.d.), 215–6.

35. Matthew Arnold, "On Translating Homer," in *On Translating Homer: With F. W. Newman's 'Homeric Translation' and Arnold's 'Last Words'* (London: George Routledge and Sons, n.d.), 6–7.

36. Paul Thompson, *The Work of William Morris* (1967; Oxford: Oxford University Press, 1993), 181; hereafter cited in text as Thompson. For a discussion of the controversy surrounding Morris and the Pre-Raphaelites and the use of an archaizing style as seen in contemporary reviews of Morris's works, see Peter Faulkner, ed., *William Morris: The Cultural Heritage* (London: Routledge & Kegan Paul, 1973). See also Gary Aho's reprint of a 1911 edition of some of Morris's early works in the archaizing style, with Aho's comprehensive introduction; William Morris, *Three Northern Love Stories and Other Tales* (Bristol: Thoemmes Press, 1996).

37. "Anglo-Saxon Leechdoms: Medicine and Astronomy in the Dark Ages," *Dublin University Magazine* 69 (May 1867): 533. What the reviewer may have meant in praising the "compactness" of the language is not entirely clear.

38. Oswald Cockayne, M.A., ed., *Hali Meidenhad: An Alliterative Homily of the Thirteenth Century* (London: Trübner, 1866), 30; hereafter referred to in text as Cockayne, *Meidenhad.*

3

The *Old English Herbarium* in a Larger European Context

It is worthwhile, therefore,
to look at the work
with an eye to its usefulness
as a medical document.
—M. A. D'Aronco and M. L. Cameron,
The Old English Illustrated Pharmacopoeia

The Herbarium of Pseudo-Apuleius *and the Early Medieval Medical Tradition*

Background and Development of the Medical Tradition

The text from which the *Old English Herbarium* was translated, the *Herbarium of Pseudo-Apuleius*, is believed to have been written in Latin as early as the fourth century.[1] It is an alphabetical treatment of medicinal plants that includes their cultivation, gathering, preparation, uses, and other information. Classical authors whose ideas can be found in the work include Dioscorides (d. A.D. 80), whose *De materia medica [The Materials of Medicine]* established a pattern for later texts; he began the tradition of mentioning the uses for a plant, how it grows, and how it could be identified.[2] Also part of the background of the *Herbarium* was Pliny the Elder, who wrote about medicinal uses of plants and about plants in general in his encyclopedic work, *Natural History*, which also served as the origin for numerous other medieval compilations.[3]

Behind the *Herbarium* as well was Galen (d. A.D. 200), the undisputed authority on medical and pharmaceutical matters throughout the Middle Ages and most of the Renaissance. Much of his treatment was based on a theory of humors in the body (blood, black bile, yellow bile, and phlegm) whose imbalance explained disease, and whose balance assured a healthy life.

Galen's writings and ideas were echoed in the *Herbarium of Pseudo-Apuleius* but were more pronounced in later medieval medicine; Galen was well known for his drug preparations, including simple medicines and mixtures using exotic ingredients, such as clays and earths from many locations around the world.[4] His writings were incorporated into many collections of medical texts, usually in part. Medical historian Jerry Stannard found that bits and pieces of Galenic theory persisted in many medieval remedies (often called *Rezepten*, mostly by Continental writers) without necessarily being linked directly to a knowledge or study of Galen: "acceptance of the doctrine of humors and its corollaries is seldom explicitly defended in the [medicinal] recipes themselves. Its defense or promulgation is usually reserved for separate, introductory chapters in leechbooks and assumed thereafter in recipes. But, as the principal explanatory basis for medical, botanical, and pharmacological theory, some form of humoralist doctrine is frequently found in recipes."[5] Examples are references in texts to hot plants, cold plants, and hot and cold conditions; many remedies are based on the concept that opposites effect cures.

However, after Dioscorides, Pliny, and Galen, no clear path leads through the medical literature of the Middle Ages, and what is today known as the *Herbarium of Pseudo-Apuleius* is actually an anonymous compilation from the fourth or early fifth century A.D. written in a Mediterranean locale. The original title is believed to have been *Herbarium Apulei Platonici traditum a Chirone Centauro, magistro Achilles.* The attribution to "Apuleius" is thought to have been added to suggest to early medieval readers that the work originated with the God of Medicine, Aesculapius.[6] The popularity of this work in the early Middle Ages is attested to in the number of surviving manuscripts from throughout Europe, many of them illustrated, and this popularity continued into the age of the printed book; it was the earliest herbal printed in Italy (1481).[7]

The late classical and early medieval world was one of flux, with peoples and boundaries in constant change; texts were copied in whole and in part, and their transmission and dissemination present huge challenges to scholars who wish to try to trace any given work to its sources.[8] Medieval medical texts developed in this milieu, and several historians have suggested that a pan-European healing tradition with a common corpus of texts, remedies, and practices best explains how to understand these texts and how they were used. In contrast to what several scholars have said about its being a classical work that was blindly copied in the Middle Ages (see the preceding chapter), the *Herbarium of Pseudo-Apuleius* appears to be an example of such a medieval text.

Very soon after the original *Herbarium* began to circulate, other works were appended and subsequently remained attached to it. For this reason, reference is sometimes made to an "enlarged" *Herbarium of Pseudo-Apuleius* (however the work is seldom if ever found without the appended texts and was considered one piece by the medieval world). The additions are *De Herba Vettonica* attributed to Antonius Musa, which is the entire first section of the *Herbarium* and lists uses for betony; *De Taxone*, which Charles Singer called a "disgusting" work on medical uses of the badger; *Medicina ex Animalibus* (or *de Quadrupedibus*) attributed to Sextus Placitus, and the *Liber medicinae ex herbis femininis*, attributed to Dioscorides.[9] Use of the fat of animals and various other parts of animals and birds in remedies was not uncommon.

As Loren MacKinney traced it, the medieval medical tradition began first in Southern France, coming out of the Roman world, and by the early Middle Ages, it was already mixed with other elements (including magic and charms) from many sources:

> The second phase of supernatural healing was a combination of pagan and Christian superstition. [The first was the early Christian emphasis on divine healing.] In Roman folk-medicine, incantations, charms, and magic played an important part. The pages of Pliny's *Natural History*, and Marcellus Empericus' handbook of medicine bear ample evidence of the fact. . . . [In spite of Christian prohibitions against things pagan] medieval folk-healers continued to use magical lore, under cover of Christian prayers and often with the sign of the cross. In similar fashion Germanic and Celtic superstitions persisted in the Christian world of medicine. (MacKinney, 28–29)

MacKinney found that the number of medical texts grew in the early Middle Ages, largely in France and Italy, but what they contained did not change appreciably, additions being wisdom supplied by practitioners as the compilations evolved over time. Apropos these texts he wrote, "Apparently those medical men who delved into the manuscripts that were available read much the same sort of material as had circulated in the West since the fifth and sixth centuries. And until the eleventh century, medical literature was to continue thus" (MacKinney, 99). It must be kept in mind that in this kind of healing the recipes and the ingredients vary widely, and substitutions are common.

The vision of a pan-European medical tradition developing in early medieval Europe is a thread that also runs throughout the articles in *Das Lorscher Arzneibuch und die frühmittelalterliche Medizin*, which brings together papers from a 1991 medical history symposium in Lorsch. The symposium centered around the Latin medical manuscript called *Das Lorscher Arzneibuch* (also known as the *Bamberger Codex*), the first medical compilation in Germany and similar in nature to the *Herbarium of Pseudo-Apuleius*. It dates to about A.D. 790 and was likely associated with the Carolingian reforms, particularly Charlemagne's ordinances known as *Capitulare* that dealt with the social good.[10]

The Lorsch contributors agreed that in the early Middle Ages, Benedictine monasteries were the major source of medical knowledge in Europe and England. Not only were medical texts like the *Herbarium of Pseudo-Apuleius* copied, excerpted, and used as references by monks who treated sick people, but the monks and their infirmaries were also a source for medical information on healing, on medicines, and on growing and collecting medicinal herbs.[11] This knowledge was passed orally and in written form from monks to other monks, to patients, and to lay persons. According to Gundolf Keil, "Monasteries established themselves as central locations for medical care in populated areas, and finally, monasteries determined to act as arbiters in transmitting the breadth and variety of the medical tradition."[12] The *Herbarium of Pseudo-Apuleius* was transmitted widely throughout the largely monastic world of healers in the early Middle Ages, as the number of surviving manuscripts attests (see Beccaria for details). In the article mentioned, Keil cited current investigations of fragmentary medical literature, the small notes and glosses about medicine that can be found in likely and unlikely places that attest to the generalized nature of medical knowledge at the time and how it was passed from person to person.

In comparing the botanical contents of classical and medieval medical texts, Stannard found that medieval *materia medica* took on a distinctive bent, tending more toward prescriptions and charms, to practical uses, than to Dioscorides's almost textbook approach to medical botany. Stannard noted that "[g]enerally speaking, much of the content of Graeco-Roman materia medica was retained but it was modified over many centuries by values, needs, and institutions of an incipient culture. One stage of the transition from ancient to medieval materia medica is represented by Marcellus of Bordeaux."[13] Stannard remarked in this article that Marcellus, a physician living in southern Gaul and writing ca. 395–410, had been generally ignored by historians of pharmacy, but studied by folklorists, notably Jacob Grimm. Marcellus's writings were a forerunner of a characteristic type of medieval medical literature, in which the names of plants were often given in two or three languages (as they are in the *Old English Herbarium*) and other elements were included, such as comments about the efficacy of the recipes, charms, and other information.

Stannard wrote about the genre:

> The change from describing medicinal plants to discussing their names is intimately connected with the development of medieval materia medica. The northward and westward expansion of European civilization away from its earlier Mediterranean homeland to the south, meant an encounter, not always quickly recognized, with a new and different flora. As a consequence, many of the locally abundant plants were unrecognized or unknown except insofar as they could be identified with the plants of the *flora classica*. Because of the

uncertainty regarding the identity, hence the properties, of these plants, names
and synonyms assumed the role formerly played by descriptions. (Stannard,
"Marcellus," 49)

In this connection, D'Aronco and Cameron said about the Old English translation of the *Herbarium*:

> The Anglo-Saxon translation observes the tradition of adding the name to a
> list of synonyms in other languages. It should however be emphasized that
> the translator chose as the key name first on the list not the name in his own
> language, but the Latin, or sometimes Greek, term for each plant. The
> Anglo-Saxon plant name was always inserted in last place, evidently
> because it was considered a kind of synonym. . . . This occurs not only in
> cases where the plants are native to the warmer zones of the Mediterranean
> basin, and therefore not necessarily common in Britain, but also for plants
> like equisetum or horsetail, found in all parts of Europe including the
> British Isles, whose English name the translator appears to be unaware of.
> (D'Aronco and Cameron, 45)

Marcellus is often said to anticipate medieval practices by including
pagan and semipagan charms, incantations, magical formulas, and charms as
intrinsic parts of the therapy, and it appears that with this kind of medical
writing, we are no longer dealing with "rational" medicine in the sense of the
classical Greek tradition, though much of it can be ultimately traced to that
source. Roman medicine, in contrast to Greek, had always included a certain
amount of what we term superstition, though Cockayne and Singer were not
careful to distinguish Greek from Roman in their concept of "classical."
Important to this argument is that Greek rational medicine very early became
part of a fluid mass of medical knowledge that was passed on in texts and
in practice, and this included charms, prayers, and rituals that were pan-
European. The *Herbarium* belonged to this tradition, not to the purely classical Greek one.

John M. Riddle, too, described a composite medical tradition in the Middle Ages, out of which works like the *Herbarium of Pseudo-Apuleius* arose.
Riddle studied the relationship between theory and practice as seen in drug
therapy ("the way most medicine was practiced") during the entire Middle
Ages. He found that both Roman and medieval medicine consisted of nonin-
stitutionalized, informal practice based on essentially the same medical education, with a medical practice that was not totally dependent on written texts
but was based on a pharmacy that preserved older knowledge and also recognized and used new drugs.[14] Riddle also argued that the movement to reestab-
lish the preeminence of medical theory from the eleventh century onward as
part of scholasticism actually produced a gap between theory and practice
because the new drug theory was unworkable. Based on a complex theoreti-

cal system involving—among other things—use of opposites to effect healing, the new remedies included more and more exotic ingredients that were
in theory supposed to work because their philosophical raisons d'être proved
they must work.

The Herbarium of Pseudo-Apuleius *as Part of* Rezeptliteratur

The *Herbarium of Pseudo-Apuleius* belongs to what is generally termed an
herbal and is also a book of remedies. An extensive body of literature is
developing on the European continent dealing with such collections of prescriptions, which are sometimes studied under the name of *Rezeptliteratur*,
and they shed light on how the *Herbarium of Pseudo-Apuleius* should be
evaluated and interpreted.[15] Sigerist was one of the few medical historians to
study in detail compilations of remedies from the early medieval period,
including the Apuleius *Herbarium*. He was a contemporary of Singer's and,
like Singer, was interested in classical medicine and its legacy. What Sigerist
sought to prove was that classical Greek medical texts survived the early
medieval period in some form and were, in fact, the foundation for the medical school at Salerno.[16] But unlike Singer, and to his credit, Sigerist meticu-
lously studied the medical literature of the late classical/early medieval
period, ca. A.D. 600–1000, to try to find the thread leading back to the Greek
medical writers, and out of this came his assessments of early medieval medical texts and their traditions. Regardless of whether his theory is valid, that
Greek medicine survived, his studies on the early medieval medical textual
traditions are extremely valuable. Sigerist wrote in 1923:

> With the end of the classical world, the darkest time began in the history of
> medical science. Galen had organized the medical knowledge of his time
> into an immense system. He stands there as the concluding piece in the
> proud structure of ancient medicine. With him concludes originality, and
> the following centuries belong to the compilers. . . . It looked even darker in
> the Latin-speaking world.[17]

In spite of his gloomy assessment, Sigerist made a meticulous study of what
was passed down in the medical texts. His studies are still extremely valuable
even if his assessment of the situation is not.

Sigerist believed that thanks to *Mönchsmedizin* [monastic medicine],
medical literature was indeed copied, but in addition, monastic and lay physicians continued to pass their craft father to son, master to apprentice (and it
might be assumed midwife to midwife as well, though he did not say so). He
also found that the classical Greek medical tradition had already begun to
include superstition. Although early medieval *Rezeptliteratur* formed the
basis for Salernitan knowledge, no two of the collections were alike, as
Sigerist described it: "The common foundation that they [the Salernitan

texts] have is nothing other than the medicinal recipe material from the sixth and seventh centuries, to which over time new remedies came or old ones in new forms" (Sigerist, *Rezeptliteratur*, 185–6).[18] The genre was in continual flux, as unusable information was thrown out and new incorporated, and new compilations were made from the old. About the genre, Sigerist concluded, "Thus I believe that in most cases we have original compilations before us, collections that the scribe assembled for the needs of his monastic/medical uses" Sigerist, *Rezeptliteratur*, 186).[19]

According to Sigerist, medical literature in the early Middle Ages could be ascribed to either a scientific tradition or to a type consisting mainly of prescriptions and originating in Pliny and Scribonius Largus. To the latter type he thought the *Herbarium of Pseudo-Apuleius* and the writings of Marcellus belonged. Agreeing with him, scholars like Riddle and Stannard also considered medical texts after the late classical era to be unique and dynamic, no matter the language in which the works were written.

Much research has been done on *Rezeptliteratur*, investigators even splitting the remedies into types. Ulrich Stoll, for example, wrote of a fundamental difference between what he termed short and long remedies, tracing the long ones to Dioscorides and Galen and their tradition, the shorter versions to the Latin world.[20] Stoll put the *Herbarium of Pseudo-Apuleius* into this genre of short remedies, that is, being early medieval and Latin. Gundolf Keil envisioned that short remedies would have been addressed to patients or to their care-givers, and that the monastery door was where medical prescriptions were passed on orally, even being translated there—and he believed this oral transmission of information was crucially important in early medieval medicine. In fact, both Keil and Stoll thought that short prescriptions, or medical bits of advice, made up most of the literature and general medical lore circulating in Europe—and in England, it might be fair to assume (see U. Stoll, and Keil and Schnitzer, "Einleitung").

The *Herbarium of Pseudo-Apuleius,* the *Old English Herbarium,* and Anglo-Saxon Medicine

The *Herbarium of Pseudo-Apuleius*, an early medieval collection of *Rezepten*, crossed the English Channel in Latin probably well before the reign of King Alfred and circulated in Anglo-Saxon England, as did numerous other Latin works. With it came a tradition of healing as it existed in the early Middle Ages—as discussed above, a practice that was disseminated orally and in writing. Many aspects of that tradition are at this point unrecoverable, but charms, incantations, and magic, as well as written texts, were very much a part of it and had been for quite some time. So were medicinal plants, many of them native not to England but to southern Europe. Cockayne was the first to bring up the Mediterranean origin of the plants in the

Herbarium, suggesting that the illustrations were therefore of no use to a reader in Great Britain. Following his suggestion, later writers have emphasized the alleged bookish nature of the *Herbarium of Pseudo-Apuleius* and the impossibility of growing many of the plants for which it calls, for these reasons alone dismissing the work as not having been useful to Anglo-Saxon healers: Why then was it translated into Old English and why were multiple manuscripts made of the translations?

When the *Herbarium of Pseudo-Apuleius* was translated into Old English (and it was probably done at least twice; see chapter 4), it was to make it more accessible to Anglo-Saxon speakers who consulted it; it was not viewed as some kind of esoteric treatise that was beyond the reach of practitioners, not the "mere" translation Singer and others deemed it. On the contrary, it was an essential text. The *Old English Herbarium* was a continuation and part of a European medieval medical tradition, just like its brothers, *Bald's Leechbook* and the *Lacnunga.* Small parts of them could be unique to Anglo-Saxon England, or to another locale, and there might be good reason for later scholars to try to isolate what may be uniquely Anglo-Saxon, but the isolated pieces become fully comprehensible only when considered as parts of a larger medical continuum—essential pieces in a large and complex puzzle.

In her study of medieval medicine, historian Nancy Siraisi saw the Old English texts in a larger, pan-European context.

> Moreover, even in regions far from the cultural and climatic conditions of the late ancient Mediterranean, early medieval copying of medical books was not divorced from practical applications. For example, the *Leechbook of Bald,* a famous medical handbook written in Old English in about the early tenth century, evidently with practical use in mind, has been shown to include numerous passages selected, translated, or adapted from Latin works; similarly, the Old English translation of the so-called *Herbal of Apuleius,* presumably a monastic or clerical endeavor, shows signs of adaptation for practical use in a local environment. (Siraisi, 10)

Linda Voigts showed specifically such an adaptation in the arrangement of the contents of the *Old English Herbarium* in her *Isis* article titled "Anglo-Saxon Plant Remedies and the Anglo-Saxons."[21]

Although they were not specifically about Anglo-Saxon England, Stannard's remarks on the development of early medieval medicine certainly did not exclude it, and in fact, in his article on Marcellus, he suggested a connection between Marcellus' writings and an Anglo-Saxon charm. That Bede might have known the writings of Marcellus was suggested by Stannard in this same article. Ogilvy too tied the bonds of learning and culture tightly between Anglo-Saxon England and the continent during the early Middle Ages, especially through the monasteries. He left no doubt that the basic texts of late classical and early medieval Europe were known to the Anglo-Saxons—including medical texts. Ogilvy traced this connection as far back as Benedict Biscop in the mid-600s: "We may be sure that so keen a bibliophile as Benedict would have observed the libraries of the monasteries he visited and must have picked up a good many books in this way by gift, purchase, or arrangement to have them copied" (Ogilvy, 5). Ogilvy said he found "overwhelming evidence for the regular sharing and transmission of books from the time of Bede forward between England and the continent" (Ogilvy, 6). One bit of evidence Ogilvy used to suggest that the Anglo-Saxons knew a certain book was the frequency of its "appearance in early Continental libraries and booklists: A work known in foundations such as St. Gall, Peronne, and Würzburg with close English connections may either have reached them from England or have been carried back to England by visitors. Students of the history of a particular work should probably pay closer attention to evidence of this sort than I have done below" (Ogilvy, 41).

Medical lore was not a static body of knowledge; as Sigerist suggested, it was in constant evolution as elements such as astrology and exotic ingredients from afar were added to the herbal prescriptions and ritual practices, and recorded knowledge reflected a variety of local needs and uses. The trend can be seen to continue, for example, in the Middle English *Agnus Castus*, a medicobotanical dictionary with alphabetical listings by the Latin name and one or more English or sometimes French names following.[22] The modern editor, Gösta Brodin, dated the *Agnus Castus* from the end of the fourteenth century and noted that it drew from Dioscorides, Hippocrates, Pliny, Galen, Isidore, and Platerius. A comparatively large number of English translations of this work exist, and even one in Welsh. Brodin said it was printed as the first part of *Bancke's Herball* in 1525, and that scattered among the recipes were thirteen charms, eight in English, four in Latin, one in French. So the tradition of borrowing, combining, and inserting helpful rituals continued well after the Apuleius per se had either disappeared or been assimilated into other works.

Although no proof exists that the *Herbarium of Pseudo-Apuleius* was translated into Old English much earlier than the eleventh century, De Vriend linked the *Old English Herbarium* to a medical tradition in England that was already old in the eleventh century.

> The study of herb medicine flourished throughout the post-classical and early medieval periods, as is abundantly proved by the survival of numerous Latin texts on the subject. There can be little doubt that these Latin treatises were studied in the Northumbrian monasteries in the seventh and eighth centuries and that the medicinal herbs were grown in the monastery gardens. The undertaking of an OE translation of a herbal in that period might be seen as a circumstance which arose as the logical result of this interest in herb medicine. (De Vriend, xlii)

He also linked the Latin manuscripts of the *Herbarium of Pseudo-Apuleius* in England (and hence the *Old English Herbarium*) to a complex manuscript tradition: "Many problems [with the manuscripts] have remained unsolved, not only because at least three originally separate texts were combined, but also because from the earliest versions onwards the manuscripts were interpolated with new material, often consisting of lists of synonyms, charms, and prayers, or personal accounts of people who had successfully used some remedy or other" (DeVriend, 1).[23] The extant manuscripts of the *Old English Herbarium* are discussed in the following chapter; four survived, attesting to the popularity of this work (and even more exist in Latin from the same period).

Linda Voigts was the first to study the *Old English Herbarium* and its illustrations in great detail, as well as the manuscript traditions to which it belongs.[24] She was also the first to question whether the Mediterranean origin of many of the medicinal plants listed in the work made the Old English and Latin herbaria more or less useless in England, as Cockayne, Singer, and others had asserted (see Voigts "Plant Remedies"). The Mediterranean origin of plants alone has fueled the argument that the *Old English Herbarium* was a "mere translation" for the Anglo-Saxons, who could not have known, much less grown, the plants. Indeed, the whole notion of a pan-European medical tradition based on similar plants could be (and has been) questioned on these grounds.

Voigts demonstrated in the article on plant remedies that many of the plants in the *Herbarium* could have been grown in Anglo-Saxon England, and not only in gardens. In fact, she showed that even if many of the plants in the *Old English Herbarium* were indeed indigenous to the Mediterranean region, this fact does not at all discount the book's usefulness in northern Europe, and in particular in England; cultivated gardens for herbs are known from the time, and it is not impossible that herbs were introduced from other regions and grown there. Voigts warned about assuming that the climate at the time the *Herbarium of Pseudo-Apuleius*, the *Old English Herbarium*, and other medical texts were written was the same as it is now for the British Isles, indeed for all of Europe. The article provides evidence to show that there was a warm period in northern Europe that lasted from the ninth to the thirteenth centuries (Voigts, "Plant Remedies," 261–3).

The point here is that many plants considered to be Mediterranean could have been grown in England (and elsewhere) during such a favorable period. But more important to this discussion is the additional fact that, using the gardening techniques that are known to have existed for monastery gardens, with care even fragile plants could have been cultivated in England no matter the weather. About this, Voigts wrote:

That the presence in England of two Mediterranean medical plants named in Anglo-Saxon remedy books seems to result from Anglo-Saxon cultivation is a crucial point for this paper and one which raises a final area of concern in the matter of Anglo-Saxon knowledge of Mediterranean plants—that of the monastic herb garden. It is important to emphasize the easily overlooked implications of the minimal climatic optimum that made cultivation of southern plants easier, but the cultivation practices bear examination in their own right. We are, after all, not so much dealing with native floral populations as with pampered plants grown within the cloister walls that radiate heat and provide shelter from the wind—plants that are weeded, mulched, and watered, in many cases annuals, for which the question of winter hardiness is irrelevant. (Voigts, "Plant Remedies," 263–64)

At least one book on medieval gardens supports Voigts's ideas. John Harvey wrote that an outstanding early record for England on gardens and gardening is Ælfric's vocabulary of 995, which he said had been disregarded because scholars contended it included names of plants and trees that could not have then been in cultivation, an argument often used to devalue the *Old English Herbarium*. However, Harvey argued that Ælfric listed words in general use in the daily conversation of the schools of Anglo-Saxon England, and that of some 200 herbs and trees he listed, only nine were doubtful of having been grown or are not easily identifiable: *wylde cyrfet, harewinta, duthhamor, eordhappel (mandragora), ficbeam (ficus), palmtwig, elebeam, unwaestmbeare elebeam, cederbeam.*[25]

The argument that gardens throughout late classical and early medieval Europe were similar south to north is strengthened by written records of what was grown and how often gardens are mentioned. There is evidence of cultivated gardens in locations as diverse as Isidore's Spain, Charlemagne's court at Aachen, the monastery at St. Gall, and Bede's England. John Harvey's volume is a comprehensive source for overview material. In his chapter two, which covers the period from 500 to 1000 A.D., he admitted the written evidence for this period was scanty, with the exception of the meticulous early ninth-century *Capitulare* from Charlemagne's court pertaining to what the emperor wanted grown in crown lands in all the imperial lands of his empire. The possible influence of Charlemagne's gardens throughout northern Europe is only hinted at in Harvey, who mentioned that King Alfred passed laws protecting vineyards and fields in England.

In addition, the avenues by which plant lore traveled throughout Europe appear to have been interwoven and complex, since the spread began in very early times and the knowledge became simply European. Archaeological evidence will reveal what was growing where and when, and whether the plants thought of as "native" really are in any one country. Lacking this evidence, as is generally the case, what is left are the medical texts with their similar plant and animal lore and a few plans for monastery or imperial gardens. For example, pushing the pan-European knowledge-base back before the medieval period, Clemens Stoll believed that the physicians who accompanied the Roman army probably managed to influence the civilian population as well, and he contended that trade, albeit severely diminished, would have continued in spite of the Romans having withdrawn to the south. As Stoll described the situation, "Classical medicine first met the Germans in battle with the Romans, especially through traders who followed the armies throughout all of Europe. Even after Rome fell, the military physicians and surgeons worked in the old Roman cities as civilians and they spread knowledge of classical medicine in the Germanic and Gallo-Celtic West."[26]

If this is true, and it seems reasonable, then it will be hard if not impossible to know when the Angles and Saxons might have learned about Mediterranean plants and the medicinal remedies based on them—possibly it was well before they came to England. Stoll also tied the monasteries of the early Middle Ages to trade: "With their knowledge and skills, and in connection with the trade and markets from Italy to the North Sea, the monasteries controlled the current stocks and important supply routes of foodstuffs, medicines, and utensils" (C. Stoll, 156).[27] The evidence is quite strong that beginning at least with Rome, the melting pot of knowledge about use of medicinal plants began its spread throughout Europe, and it simply continued.

To complicate the picture of plant life in the United Kingdom, Miles Hadfield cited conditions that still prevail in the western regions that allow flora from diverse foreign soils to thrive:

> Perhaps the most remarkable feature of our landscape climate from the gardener's point of view is that along our western seaboard—from Cornwall to Loch Ewe in the north of Scotland—are many districts where plants and trees from such diverse places as the Pacific Coast of North America, western China, Tibet, and the Himalayas, New Zealand and Chile thrive in the moist, windy, but temperate air.[28]

Records for the early medieval monastery at St. Gall in today's Switzerland provide details about the plan for medieval monasteries and they date from approximately the same era as Charlemagne's decrees on gardens. The monastery plan of about 816–820 A.D. shows an infirmary and an infirmary garden (the *Herbularius*) on which the names of the plants are written: kidney bean, savory, rose, mint, cumin, lovage, fennel, tansy or costmary, lily, sage, rue, flag iris, pennyroyal, fenugreek, and rosemary (Harvey, 32–3). In addition to this medicinal garden, the monastery had a kitchen garden and an ornamental orchard, which also served as the monastery cemetery.

Voigts's article on plant remedies, using St. Gall as one example, is again instructive:

> Two other observations on the improvement of the Pseudo-Apuleius remedy book should be made. At Saint Gall a ninth-century herbal survives which seems to have originated there (Stiftsbibliothek, 217). It contains entries for sixty-two plants. Thirty-six of the chapters derive from the

> *Herbarium Apulei*, but twenty-six have no known source, and a number of
> those seem to be the addition of alpine plants. . . . It may also be significant
> that the *Ex herbis femininis* treatise which accompanies the Pseudo-
> Apuleius herbal in the Old English texts seems to be a sophisticated
> reworking of Dioscoridean materials by someone in Ostrogothic Italy who
> knew the plants in the treatise. (Voigts, "Plant Remedies," 256)

From the scattered but not inconsiderable evidence throughout early-medieval Europe, it is clear that cultivation of gardens was usual, particularly for plants valued for medicinal uses, and that the same or similar plants were grown pretty much everywhere. Those that could not be grown seem to have been traded (see Voigts, "Plant Remedies," 266). It is also clear that the *Herbarium of Pseudo-Apuleius* was a reference work popular throughout western Europe, including England, where it was used in Latin and as the *Old English Herbarium* as a practical guide to medicinal plants, their use, and remedies to be made with them. The plants were available, either grown in gardens and stored, or traded, and they were familiar to people throughout Europe.

Using Living Traditions of Healing to Comprehend Medieval Medicine

To understand how a partially unwritten body of knowledge about plants and healing survived fairly intact over many centuries and in many geographical locales, the living, ancient *curandera* (folk-healer) tradition of the southwestern United States not only serves as a model, but its roots can be traced to the medieval herbal tradition under discussion. Indeed, the modern practice of herbal medicine has the same roots. Marta Weigle and Peter White wrote in *The Lore of New Mexico*, "[In Hispanic villages consulted in 1959–60], specialized therapists were the *partera*, or midwife; the *médica/-o* or *yerbera/-o*, who has herbal expertise; the *sobador/-a*, or massager, who also knows skin snapping or sometimes cupping, or *ventosa*, the use of suction to draw out pain; and the *curandera/-o*, who is more often female and who can deal with many kinds of illness, including witchcraft."[29] Weigle said that the *curandera* used medical treatment (mainly herbal) and religious rites, such as prayers and appeals to saints, and attempts to set right again causes of imbalances or sources of bewitchments; however her concentration was more on witchcraft and miraculous healing than healing with plants. *Curandera* (f) is used here to represent the tradition because she is more common, though *curandero* (m) or *curanderismo* would do.

The *curandera*—a healer using herbs and ritual—came to the New World from medieval Spain with remedies from Europe and even Morocco. Through the years, the tradition picked up information and ingredients from indigenous populations in the New World, and added even more to the stock of information as settlers moved into the southwestern regions of the United States beginning in about 1500. The medical tradition she came from in Europe included university-trained physicians and folk healers who practiced at the same time, but in different social strata, and the colonizers of New Mexico were not the upper class, by and large. The medicinal ingredients for all healers was essentially the same no matter the social class, yet university-trained physicians tended to use expensive imports along with the common herbs.

The medical background in Spain was described by Siraisi, who was writing about late medieval and Renaissance physicians and healers.

> [By the late thirteenth and fourteenth centuries] University graduates in medicine occupied the highest place, followed by other skilled medical practitioners, then by skilled surgeons, and finally by barber surgeons and various other practitioners, among them herbalists or apothecaries. Some form of this hierarchy was to be found in most parts of western Europe, although in various regions university graduates in medicine were a rarity before the late fifteenth century; everywhere the hierarchy involved a good deal of social as well as occupational stratification. . . . Members of the medical profession thus varied widely in training, type of formal qualification (if any), occupation, and social and economic status. *Yet, despite this diversity, they shared a common medical culture* in which they participated with differing degrees of intellectualization and sophistication. Hence, delineation of the general contours of medical activity in broad and nonrestrictive terms will promote an understanding of the uses to which medical knowledge was put as well as the impact of new forms of medical knowledge as they became diffused in a variety of ways and at many different levels [emphasis added]. (Siraisi, 20 and 23. Her chapter "Practitioners and Conditions of Practice" covers this topic in detail.)

No small part of the common medical culture was the body of knowledge, written and unwritten, about medicinal plants, which made its inexact way through the hands and words of many during the course of two millennia—and which promises to continue. For example, there is evidence that Phillip II of Spain provided funds to Francisco Hernandez, one of his physicians, to go to New Spain in 1570 to record the plants—the *materia medica*—and animals of the New World. Hernandez based his information on a written Aztec codex and on exhaustive interviews with local inhabitants and one personal experience with the drugs. The outcome was his *Rerum Medicarum Novae Hispaniae Thesaurus*, which had an unhappy subsequent history. But the point here is that, along with a search for gold, the old world was looking at the new for a new pharmacopoeia, presumably in plant form.

An appeal to the living and changing *curandera* tradition in the southwestern United States as it is practiced today lends credibility to the argument that by considering the presence of a common, largely unwritten, and constantly evolving tradition of healing during late classical and early medieval periods in Europe, the medical tradition of those times can be better understood. The *curandera* tradition is appropriate to cite here because of its similarities to the medieval one, because of its roots in medieval Europe, and because the situation under which it began in the United States (then a Spanish territory) shows remarkable similarities to the situation in Anglo-Saxon England, or for that matter to most of Europe during late classical and early medieval times. It was a world where peoples were conquered, sometimes repeatedly, merged with the conquerors or migrated into unfamiliar locales and adapted, taking much with them and learning the new.[30] The medical knowledge that any healer had, whether barbarian, Roman colonial, Anglo-Saxon leech, or Spanish *curandera*, was largely passed down from person to person and it was based on knowledge of the use of plants for the most part—this can be traced in the texts. Ritual was part of healing from the earliest days. When familiar plants were not available, new ones with a similar appearance or smell were tried. In New Mexico, local Pueblo Indians shared their medical lore and plants with the Spanish settlers of Mexico.[31]

As mentioned above, Clemens Stoll argued quite plausibly that a similar situation prevailed throughout Europe from the time of Christ: the Roman army and its entourage bringing plants, texts, physicians, the conquered people picking up some of this knowledge and adding to their own healing lore, then being themselves trained and combining old knowledge with new and passing it on. It would have been the same with the medieval monks and their medicine. In fact Stoll described how medical training occurred in the monasteries, and it is markedly similar to today's *curandera*'s apprenticeship:

> With regard to the multiplicity of remedies, the imprecision of the nomenclature, and the uncertainty in measurements, the question arises concerning the scientific and practical knowledge of the monks who were responsible for preparing the medications. The practical skills and experience could only have been gained during a long period in a monastic pharmacy (where medicines are prepared), such as the pharmacies shown in the plans for monasteries during the Carolingean period. *This knowledge would have been transmitted personally from one monk to another.* Above all, the itinerant Irish monks, for whom the monasteries on the Continent served as havens, for example St. Gall, Lorsch, or Reichenau, spread that kind of knowledge from their home monasteries [emphasis added]. (C. Stoll, 178)[32]

The monasteries and monks of Anglo-Saxon England were part of this European-wide system of healing, where apprenticeship, word-of-mouth information, trading, and texts all contributed to the healer's art. The not inconsiderable slave population throughout Europe, which brought men, women, and children onto alien soils, might have also influenced disseminating plants and knowledge of plants and could have contributed to the general medical lore as well.

The person-to-person distribution of medical knowledge that existed in colonial New Spain persists in New Mexico (to cite one instance of how this tradition was kept alive). About the tradition, Michael Moore, a recognized specialist in the herbal tradition of the Southwest, wrote:

> The New Mexican, either indio, primo, or anglo, is surrounded by plants whose medicinal uses are known and systematized by hundreds and thousands of years of usage. The remedios in this little book are a complete hybrid of two cultures. The spanish primos brought their traditional herbs, such as Manzanilla and Alhucema; the pueblo indians introduced them to Inmortal and Osha. Present usage is the result of nearly four hundred years of Spanish and over a thousand years of Indian pragmatism. . . . What I have compiled in this book is what I have learned, observed and used as of 1977, a frozen cross-section of a moving stream.[33]

In the book, similar to medieval medical texts, Moore listed the Spanish, Latin, and English names for the plants and their primary and secondary uses.

Moore's observations were corroborated at a week-long seminar on "Medicinal Plants of the Southwest" held at Ghost Ranch, New Mexico, in June 1997, taught by three practicing herbalists who gather their plants in the wild and obtain them from commercial sources. As the workshop leaders pointed out, for anyone, yesterday and today, who collects plants in the wild, as opposed to growing or obtaining them from another, a difficult part of the task is simply being able to identify the plants in the field. Even armed with a modern field guide to herbs and with photos and drawings, identification is often only made possible by familiarity with the plant itself. Sometimes only a slight difference is crucial; for example, the slightly sticky feel of a true cleavers, which has medicinal properties, is all that distinguishes it from a nonmedicinal and similar-looking brother growing nearby. All three of the workshop leaders operated from a similar body of knowledge about herbs and plants and ingredients used in preparing them, but each one had slight variations on what might be prescribed for a given condition, or differed in opinion on the best remedy for another. A strategy of starting with a small dose to see what works and being willing to alter the remedy was the rule, as was the most important ingredient—patience. Unlike chemical medicines, herbs (poisonous ones excepted) do not usually work immediately.

Apropos identification of plants in the field and how herbal medicine works, in *Magic and Medicine of Plants*, intended to be a practical guide to seeking, growing, using, and understanding the long history of medicinal plants, the editors wrote:

Sometimes even a botanist may be baffled by a plant that seems to be a member of a certain species, but has some characteristics that are not typical. Or a collector may identify a certain plant in a region where authoritative sources say it has never grown before. It happens for a number of reasons. First, no two individual plants look exactly alike. They can vary in height, leaf shape and size, flower color, or any of a number of other characteristics. This phenomenon, called biological variation, is the result of differences in the genetic makeup of individuals. . . . As for plants in the "wrong" place, similar environments may be hundreds or even thousands of miles apart, but if a plant from one somehow manages to reach the other—naturally or through human intervention—it has a good chance of taking hold in the new area. As one botanist remarked, some plants "have never read the book" defining what their habitat and range should be.[34]

Familiarity with the flora and familiarity with families of plants are thus essential to the tradition of gathering plants to use medicinally (or for food, for that matter): Texts are only a reminder. Such must have been the case with the medieval medical texts, whose illustrations have long been considered worthless in identifying the plants to which they refer. It is possible, indeed probable, that the illustrations were never intended to be any kind of field guide, but served as aids to memory. After all, plants look different at different points in their growing cycle, and one picture (or drawing) captures it at one point in its life. Plant illustration in manuscripts and books is a study with which specialists grapple, as seen for example in Heide Grape-Albers, *Spätantike Bilder aus der Welt des Arztes: Medizinische Bilderhandschriften der Spätantike und Ihre Mittelalterliche Überliferund*,[35] in Minta Collins's *Medieval Herbals*,[36] in Voigts's dissertation, and in the D'Aronco and Cameron facsimile of the *Old English Herbarium*. However these works do not discuss illustrated medieval medical manuscripts from the standpoint of their usefulness to a healer, rather they trace illustrative traditions throughout Europe in an effort to connect manuscript stemma. In fact, the human figures at the beginning of the Cotton MS receive far more scholarly attention than the plant illustrations. The plant illustrations deserve further study to determine their usefulness in identifying plants and preparing the listed remedies. Granted they are not lifelike, but undoubtedly they served a purpose other than decoration.

The usefulness of the illustrations has been questioned because they are not what we consider to be realistic. The possible efficacy of the remedies has been questioned on much the same grounds. Several medicinal plants in the *Herbarium* are suggested to help heal the same condition, but no guidelines are given on how to choose one. The modern world does not like such imprecision. Here the practice of herbology can help in understanding the medieval text. All the listed plants may help either alone or with other plants, and experienced healers who know the plants have their own preferred cures.

They do not require detailed instructions. Writing about preparation of such medicines in the medieval world, C. Stoll said:

> To the almost countless numbers of simples [remedies using one plant], early medieval medicine added a large choice of composites [remedies using several plants]. Here, the monks served to organize and collect the texts that had been scattered and then they made them useful for and accessible to the monasteries. . . . The early medieval monks took antidotes and remedies from classical works and often adapted them to local and personal needs, for which reason hardly any of the anonymous collections of remedies agrees fully with another. (C. Stoll "Arznei," 175–76)[37]

Illuminating to the topic here is Stoll's point that many of the preparations differ ever so slightly from one compilation to another, even though they used similar ingredients for similar treatments. And particularly significant is the fact that substitutions were commonly made for ingredients, using a plant or other ingredient with similar properties, a trend seen in the later Middle Ages in extensive lists of possible quid pro quo substitutions. This same practice was seen to be alive and well in the course of a nine-month class titled "Foundations of Herbalism" at the National College of Phytotherapy in Albuquerque, New Mexico, in 1998–99, which became the North American College of Botanical Medicine in 2000.

Regarding the *curandera* tradition and the use of herbs in New Mexican folk medicine, Curtin's *Healing Herbs of the Upper Rio Grande* features a foreword by novelist and folklorist Mary Austin, a longtime resident of Santa Fe. In it, an additional element of plant and medical knowledge in the Southwest is brought out:

> Here is [in herbalism of the Southwest], first of all, the tribal approach in which there is free play of the experimental method of discovery; there is also the folk method which consists of tradition explicitly touched by the early phases of the doctrine of signatures, marked by racial crossings and migrations, such as included the intrusion of Moorish practice transferred to Spain and from Spain to America, with overlappings of traditional Indian, Spanish, and Moorish lore. By such migrations the reach of botanical experience has been expanded not only by extensions of the known field, but also by the substitutions of one familiar remedy for another which in another environment it greatly resembled, and the crossings of mingling traditions.[38]

The situation in New Mexico, with its mingling of cultures and a sharing of information in whatever form available, written or from memory, does not differ appreciably from what is written about early medieval Europe. The difficulty on this level—person to person, often both unlettered—is that no record remains of their transactions and conversations. The outcome, years later, of these transactions may be the only witness to their having occurred. The slight changes in copies and versions of medieval medical texts witness to much unrecorded information altered by human interactions over the course of many years in many countries, and help explain how the common reservoir of knowledge about healing and plants was spread both by texts and in person. Curtin described it in this somewhat romanticized way:

> Faith and fatalism are the first ingredients in folk medicine; under these is the tradition of properties, and the trail of tradition is sometimes long and winding. Here, for example, is *alfilerillo* (filaree), brought from across the seas with its Moorish name, growing wild as native weed but treasured still for its helpful attributes. From Mexico, too, have come names and uses learned from the Aztec, and not a little knowledge has accrued from a long and friendly intercourse with the local Pueblo Indians. Such are the exigencies of sickness in a land without doctors that the memories of the people must be stored with the harvest of centuries. (Curtin, 12)

Source studies, searches for *motifs*, the isolation of the barbarian from the classical in medieval medical texts, specifically in the triad of Anglo-Saxon texts, have value as evidence for what actually happened *in the texts*. But written evidence only captures part of the healing tradition in the early medieval period. The reason that changes occurred in medical manuscripts as they were translated or copied may actually have stemmed from Cameron's "common body of knowledge" and the monks and other practitioners' interpreting rather than blindly translating. Current efforts to understand the actual practice of medicine in medieval Europe are approaching the subject in such a critical manner, with studies on how herbal and other remedies as found in the manuscripts actually work.

The *Old English Herbarium* as a Practical Medical Text

In the belief that the *Old English Herbarium* (and by extension the Latin *Herbarium of Pseudo-Apuleius* and similar medieval medical texts) was valuable to healers in Anglo-Saxon England and could be used if properly understood, the present study is not exclusively based on texts, but includes practical experience with the modern tradition of herbology, which is based on medicinal plants and whose foundation includes medieval *herbaria* and works like them.[39] Undertaking such a practical study was suggested, if indirectly, by the new approaches to Anglo-Saxon medicine in particular and medieval medicine generally that are cited here, but especially by the groundbreaking work of Voigts, Riddle, Cameron, D'Aronco, and Bart Holland. The *Old English Herbarium* is clearly a text with meaningful, if cryptic, content; to understand it is no mystery, but essential to understanding the cryptography is knowledge of how herbal medicine is practiced and how its remedies are made, much like understanding a terse recipe by being able to cook.

Such an approach is found in "A drynke þat men callen dwale to make a man to slepe whyle men kerven him: A surgical anesthetic from late Medieval England." Here, Voigts and Hudson reported on their study of numerous Middle English manuscripts in which they sought evidence that surgical anesthetics were used and also, when found, the ingredients they contained. Although the article is about recipes for an anesthetic called *dwale,* which the authors have found in at least twenty-seven different Middle English manuscripts, it illustrates well the new, more scientific approach to the contents of medieval and Renaissance herbals and recipe books. About their approach, the authors wrote:

> We also think it helpful to draw on the resources of twentieth-century pharmacological knowledge to analyze the recipe [for *dwale*]. It must be understood, however, that the use of current pharmacological literature has distinct limitations when applied to texts like *dwale.* Pharmacology today involves a high degree of accuracy in identification and quantification that cannot exist for medieval medicinal compounds. Indeed, nineteenth-century dispensatories are more useful for studying medieval medicine than are today's textbooks of pharmacology. Older dispensatories provide details of pharmacognosy, medical indications, methods of preparation, warnings, dosages, and so on that no longer appear in current descriptions of highly standardized, often synthetic medicaments.[40]

The ingredients were analyzed in turn, including what each was mixed with, to find out whether such a recipe would work in producing sleep, and if so why. The authors cited a similar approach by M. L. Cameron, who had, for example, examined a text long thought to be magic because it prohibited the use of iron. Cameron looked at the recipe not as a magical text, but from the standpoint of a scientist, questioning whether using an iron container would have affected the ingredients in any way. The answer was yes, and the recipe was found to be based on observation and experience. Such was Voigts's and Hudson's approach here. A careful study of the ingredients and the instructions on how to administer the drink as well as the details about how to awaken the patient (use vinegar and salt on the temples) led them to the conclusion that this Middle English *stupefactive,* as it was called, did work and that the ingredients were carefully prescribed and thought out. An interesting conclusion they reached was that this may well have been an English invention; soporific sponges were the rule on the Continent and *dwale* was the only native English name for a medicinal recipe found in Middle English texts.

The approach taken by Voigts and Hudson supports the present approach of using the *curandera* and modern traditions of herbal medicine to shed light on how medieval medicine was actually practiced, given the medieval texts and their lack of precision in dosage and the uncertainty of the plant or plants that could be administered for a given condition. Imprecision is actually not a negative aspect of traditional herbal remedies, medieval or modern; they draw their strength from the healer's knowledge about the patient and the observed symptoms, and about the available plants and recipes that might help. Again from the article on *dwale*:

> What we cannot know, of course, is the dosage. The recipe, which says the patient should drink until he falls asleep, is vague on that point, but that vagueness may be deliberate. Even if we assume that the names in the recipe correspond to current terminology, several factors underscore the possible variations in a medieval recipe. We cannot identify the plant species with certainty, and the time and method of collection and the preparation all result in variations in the amount of active ingredient present. It is almost certain that large differences in amounts of active ingredients were the rule, a situation that is emphasized repeatedly in the twentieth century. Adding to these uncertainties are the idiosyncratic reactions to drugs and anesthetics that still vex medicine today. . . . All these variables, over which the medieval medical practitioner has no control, suggest that the practice of giving *dwale* until the patient fell asleep was undoubtedly safer than giving some prescribed amount. (*Dwale*, 42)

John Riddle, like Voigts, showed that many of the medieval remedies can be proven to work. His "Theory and Practice in Medieval Medicine" (cited earlier) and his many other published works treat medieval remedies in a practical manner. For example, he wrote: "Although speculative medical theory was almost totally abandoned, fifth-century through tenth-century records show that medical progress was not solely dependent on written language. Instead this evidence shows that a medical practice existed based upon a pharmacy that not only preserved the older practical knowledge but also recognized and used new drugs" (Riddle, "Theory," 159).

Particularly relevant to the argument advanced here—that oral as well as written transmission of knowledge occurred over many years in medieval Europe and in the early centuries of the New World—is Riddle's remark: "The texts of medieval pharmaceutical treatises generally are less descriptive of the herbs and minerals than classical texts, and thus require that the reader have some prior acquaintance with the subject before using the written words" (Riddle, "Theory," 163). He described the way in which this information was transmitted:

When one particular part of an herb, say a root, was found as being effective for some specific action, this information was orally transmitted whenever and wherever men communicated and one generation taught the other. This process takes place independently of literary transmission. There was a continuous practice of medicine which was independent of loss, attrition, or, eventually, the recovery of classical medical theory. Far from being a gray science in a gray, confused period, early medieval medicine was a partly empirical skill. . . . The assumption that one can know early medieval medicine simply in identifying the texts is faulty. (Riddle, "Theory," 165)

Riddle found witnesses to interest in medicine even in the early Middle Ages and in very widespread places, such as in Visigothic and Ostrogothic law codes, in tenth-century Welsh laws, and in Norse medicine, which he said "shows absorption of classical and southern European medicine even before Christian conversion" (Riddle, "Theory," 166). In addition, he pointed to evidence, such as King Alfred's often-quoted remark about wishing to obtain hard-to-find ingredients from the East, for a continuous drug trade between the eastern and western Mediterranean worlds.

A strong advocate for studying scientifically the possible efficacy of medieval remedies, M. L. Cameron said that a quarter of the drugs used in medicine today are from flowering plants or are synthetic and copy products made from plants, adding:

Much evaluation of plants and their medicinal value is now in progress in pharmaceutical laboratories and the results are often of much interest. The greater part of the identifiable ingredients of the Anglo-Saxon pharmacopoeia are still to be found in herbal collections and are used for the same purposes, so that we may say that Anglo-Saxon remedies were probably as good as those recommended by herbalists today. Moreover, a surprisingly large number of their ingredients are known from recent investigation to contain substances of real therapeutic value and to have been used by them for conditions where their therapeutic value should have had beneficial effects . . . as good as anything available up to the end of the nineteenth century.[41]

Cameron, a botanist, went into some detail not only about the medicinal qualities of some of the plants, but into the quite rational and scientific basis for many of the directions in preparing the remedies in the three Anglo-Saxon medical texts. For example, a remedy for eye infection that Storms attributed to the realm of magic, Cameron showed to be the result of careful observation:

Celandine is the greater celandine (*Chelidonium majus*); it exudes a bright orange latex from all injured parts. This latex in the fresh state is a powerful irritant, but after drying or heating, the irritant property is much reduced or destroyed. In this state it has been used since time immemorial to remove films or spots from the cornea of the eye. Copper salts and honey are bactericidal. The remedy [in *Bald's Leechbook*, but also found in the *Herbarium* and in Dioscorides] may have been of some help for a bacterial infection of the eye complicated by spotting or filming of the cornea. But why the warning in the Old English recipe about warming the preparation "skillfully"? Honey and celandine juice are both rather thick liquids and so burn easily when heated. This explains the need for a gentle fire and for extreme care in the cooking. Someone along the way in the preparation of this recipe thought it important to give warning of these problems. (Cameron, 121)

Cameron's arguments can also be used to debunk some of the findings of magic in the remedies; he assumed everything in a medicinal recipe might have had a rational basis and tried to find it before assuming it was magic or superstition, and he analyzed several medieval prescriptions. For example, when a recipe called for preparations either in or with copper or brass, Cameron explained this was necessary because the ingredients would react with the metal to form copper salts, which destroy all living cells, including bacteria. Also, using such antibiotic agents as onion or garlic mixed with acidic liquids such as wine or gall, the medieval remedies would have been effective against bacteria in infections, Cameron found. It is clear even from the limited number of ancient and medieval remedies that Cameron studied that many of them contain valuable information about possible uses for medicinal plants and about the rationale behind the way preparations were to be made. Particularly important is his admonition that it is dangerous to assume anything is a "magic" element in a recipe simply because it may not appear rational to the modern mind. In fact, Cameron questioned assumptions about certain charms long held to be pagan, and he found in many instances magical—often Christian—elements were added to rational formulas, making the whole formula seem magical to a modern reader.

John Mann, professor of organic chemistry at Reading, demonstrated in a recent work the scientific basis for many folk remedies, a number of which are herbal. He wrote, "The remedies that we buy are often the same as those which were prescribed 5000 years ago. The same can be said for many of the medicines we use, and the aim of this book is to demonstrate how at least some of the substances used for murder, magic, and folk medicine have been successfully transformed into clinically acceptable drugs."[42]

Mann's discussion of the science of pharmacology and his examples of specific herbs are to the point and informative, yet he was careful always to point out the negative aspects of the era and to indicate that people actually believed in charms and elves. Mann's sketch of the development of medieval medicine was this:

The barbarian invasions heralded the Dark Ages in Europe (the fifth to eleventh centuries) and herbal knowledge was kept alive initially through the works of scribes in Constantinople, then in the libraries of the rapidly expanding Arab empire. . . . Meanwhile, during the Dark Ages in Europe, pharmacy, superstition, and magic became inextricably intertwined. A number of "leechbooks" (from the Anglo-Saxon *laece*, to heal) were compiled, containing some recognizable drugs, but mostly fanciful brews for fending off elves and goblins. The most famous of these leechbooks is undoubtedly the Leechbook of Bald. . . . Even a cursory examination of this leechbook leaves one in no doubt that Bald and his contemporaries believed explicitly in the existence of elves and goblins. According to Bald, disease was primarily due to "elf-shot" or "flying venom," and his herbal brews were both protective and curative. (Mann, 114–15)

Mann did not cite Singer, Cockayne, or any contemporary scholars who have studied and published on medieval medicine; however, the positive aspect of his work is that his approach looks favorably at the long tradition of healing with herbs and other plants, at least from the standpoint of whether and how they actually work. On the other hand, he is negative toward medieval medical practice generally.

In contrast, Bart K. Holland, an epidemiologist and pharmaceutical researcher at the New Jersey School of Medicine, took the old texts quite seriously. In fact he suggested they were good sources for as-yet undiscovered modern drugs and called for collaboration between pharmacy and literature. In his *Prospecting for Drugs in Ancient and Medieval European Texts: A Scientific Approach*, Holland said:

It seems clear to me that the field of pharmaceutical sciences would stand to benefit if the "keepers of the texts" and the "keepers of the laboratories" were to increase their mutual awareness. As a medical school faculty member involved in the management of clinical trials, I have had conversations with pharmacologists who were unaware of the very large numbers of Greek and Latin medical texts, and unaware of their accessibility. I have heard such questions as, "Are there still people around who know (or can read) these works? Where do you find copies?"[43]

The book was an outgrowth of an earlier article that appeared in the magazine, *Nature,* where Holland wrote:

The scientific revolution which began in the mid-sixteenth century dismissed Aristotelian-Galenic medicine as being fraught with errors and as having a stifling influence. This attitude has persisted, causing us to regard ancient and mediaeval medicine as an historical curiosity rather then a source of potential therapies. . . . Perhaps the time has come to make a relatively small investment in the systematic re-examination of therapies mentioned in Greek and Latin medical texts, through a dialogue between pharmacologists on the one hand and historians of medicine on the other.

Such cooperation, which would link ancient texts with modern standards of testing, might result in a useful and inexpensive source of potentially therapeutic compounds.[44]

A chapter in Holland's book is devoted to the process needed to go "From Plant Lore to Pharmacy," using a well-defined process that the National Cancer Institute developed and used in the 1960s and 1970s in a search for cancer cures based on plants. The author, Thurman Hunt of the New Jersey School of Medicine, called first of all for identifying a plant in an ancient (or medieval) text that seemed worthy of investigation, then seeking ethnobotanical information to verify and clarify the information—an approach that would be interesting in coupling a work like the *Herbarium* and the *curandera* tradition of the Southwest, since both belong to the same medieval European tradition of healing. Hunt wrote:

Once a prospective plant has been identified from an ancient text, how do we verify its effectiveness and subsequently make it available for use as a pharmaceutical agent in the United States and other countries? First, we start by matching the plant's medicinal uses found in ancient texts with currently available ethnobotanical information. . . . For years modern ethnobotanists have collected and catalogued the medicinal uses of thousands of plant species. These data can be compared with the data obtained from ancient texts in order to identify any areas of overlap. This process, although often laborious, can offer many clues and lend strength and credibility to a lead which originated from a medieval or other historical source.[45]

Clearly then, medieval remedies should first be taken at face value, and nothing in them assumed to be magic or fanciful (modern physicians do not totally discount prayer or charms if they help the patient believe he will be cured). When the texts are studied as valuable witnesses to past medical practice, it is possible that even today some new information can be gleaned.

Evaluating the Remedies in the Old English Herbarium

Whether a remedy in the *Old English Herbarium* can be proved scientifically to work is a matter for the pharmaceutical researchers to determine. However, it can be shown that the plants in the *Herbarium* could have been grown, obtained, and used in Anglo-Saxon England, and thus, the work for that reason should not be said to have been useless for its time. It does not represent some kind of higher medical knowledge beyond the reach of the monks, midwives, and leeches of the time. The majority of the remedies in the *Herbarium* could have been prepared with no esoteric ingredients or equipment, and they, like those in Dioscorides, like those in the sixteenth-century Culpepper's *Herbal*, and like those in scores of twentieth-century publications are based on simple methods of preparation and generally on a plant or plants and a few other fairly common ingredients. Granted, however, medieval ingredients may not always be common now in our modern urban environment.

As is apparent from the translation in chapter 5, the preparations in the *Old English Herbarium* are actually quite simple. The numbers in parentheses behind the excerpts below refer to chapters in the *Herbarium*, standard in every edition. The translations here are the author's:

> For liver disturbances, pick some vervain on Midsummer's day, and crush it into a powder; take five spoonfuls of the powder and three draughts of good wine; mix them together and give to the patient to drink. (4)
>
> For a headache, take some basil, crush it with rose or myrtle juice [probably the essence of these plants] or vinegar and put it on the forehead. (19)
>
> [Rue] Soak the leaves in old wine, then put the extract into a glass container; afterwards apply it. [Dioscorides has a whole chapter on wines used in medicines.] Pound the rue in a wooden bowl, then pick up as much as you can grasp with three fingers, put it into a container and add a draught of wine mixed with two draughts of water, then give it as a drink . . . (117)
>
> For sores, mix together leeks, lard, bread and coriander as you would to make a poultice, and put the mixture on the sore. (125)

The reference to Midsummer's day in remedy 4 has been said to be a bit of magic, but most probably it indicates when the plant is best to harvest.

The remedies in the *Old English Herbarium* call for seething, boiling, and mixing plants with fats and waxes, crushing and chopping them, drying them, and making decoctions and teas, to name but a few of the procedures. In the twentieth century, Grieve's *A Modern Herbal* gives the following quite similar directions for medicinal remedies.

> An infusion may be made by pouring a pint of boiling water on an ounce of the bruised root [of angelica] and two tablespoonfuls of this should be given three or four times a day, or the powdered root administered in doses of 10 to 30 grains. (38)
>
> Black Bryony is a popular remedy for removing discoloration caused by bruises and black eyes, etc. The fresh root is scraped to a pulp and applied in the form of a poultice. For sores, old writers recommend it being made into a ointment with "hog's grease or wax, or other convenient ointment." (131)[46]

By appealing to the still-living tradition of herbal treatment, it can be seen that the preparations do not vary much from their presentation more than a thousand years ago. For example, *Jeanne Rose's Herbal* includes directions for gathering, storing, and using medicinal plants that are similar to those included in medieval remedies:

It is important to handle plants gently and properly. Never handle them with
a metal object unless it is a magic sword. Always use wood, enamel, glass,
or stoneware to contain and cook them in. The only metal that should touch
them is the knife or scissors used to sever the plants, or the leaves or bark
from the rest of the plant. . . . Leaves should be collected in clear, dry
weather, in the morning after the dew is gone and the sun is not yet high.
The aromatic oils are at their greatest strength at this time. . . . Barks are
gathered in the fall or the spring when the plant is at least two years old. The
bark should be dried and allowed to age for about two years before using.
(123–24) [This prohibition against metal was also given in the Ghost Ranch
class on medicinal plants mentioned earlier.]

You don't need any special equipment for making your own teas and
ointments. An enamel or glass pot, a strainer, wooden spoons, paper towels,
and a hanging type postal scale will do; you probably have all you need in
your kitchen. (125)[47]

Directions are included on how to make teas, infusions, decoctions, tinc-
tures, elixirs, essences, ointments and salves, plasters, poultices, syrups, and
cerates (126–27); they are the same procedures for making preparations as in
the *Old English Herbarium*, *Bald's Leechbook*, and countless other early
medieval remedy books and herbals. And they are the same as found in works
written about southwestern herbal medicine as practiced by the *curanderas*.

[Hediondilla or Chapparal Bush] Primary: a poultice for rheumatism.
Method A: Slowly pan fry the leaves in lard, cool, and apply. Method B:
Grind with Osha and Tobacco, mix with beeswax or Trementina, warm and
apply. A pint of the leaves can be boiled in a gallon of water for an hour and
used in a bath. Remain until the water is cool; not recommended more than
once every several months. (Moore, 10)

[Moradilla or Dakota Vervain] . . . the powdered tops can be mixed
with lard or vaseline and applied to the back of the neck for pain. (Moore,
12)

The *Old English Herbarium* in a New Context

The preface to the *Old English Herbarium* that Cockayne wrote in the Rolls
Series paints a negative picture of medieval medicine generally and casts
doubts about the usefulness of the *Herbarium* to the Anglo-Saxon world.
And yet evidence shows that the *Old English Herbarium* and the work on
which it was based, the Latin *Herbarium of Pseudo-Apuleius*, were important and serious texts for early to late medieval healers. For this reason, it is
important to the history of medicine to understand their place in the development of a medieval tradition of healing. To place the *Old English Herbarium*
into a narrow category of being in a classical or rational tradition, that is,
based on Greek theory and existing largely in the world of books, does not do

it justice. Evidence points to its having been part of a rich, varied, and unique early medieval tradition that was similar throughout Europe. Evidence also suggests that the *Herbarium*—in Latin and Old English—would have been useful and used in Anglo-Saxon England. The preparations are not difficult or esoteric, and the ingredients could have been grown, collected, or imported. It appears that lay and monastic practitioners were part of the early medical tradition, with some of the information transmitted in texts, some orally. This kind of transmission is markedly similar to the *curandera* lore of the Southwest, a healing tradition that began in medieval Spain and came to the New World, where it mingled with Native American practices. It is also the way a good deal of practical wisdom is today transmitted, together with textbook information, by modern herbologists. The modern translation offered in chapter 5 opens the *Herbarium* to a much wider audience than literary specialists, particularly those interested in the still-living practice of herbology and medical historians.

Notes

1. Hubert Jan De Vriend, *The Old English Herbarium and Medicina de Quadrupedibus*, EETS, O.S. 286 (London: Oxford University Press, 1984), lvii; hereafter cited in text as De Vriend. See also Ernst Howald and H. E. Sigerist, *Antonii Musae de Herba Vettonica Liber, Pseudo-Apulei Herbarius, Anonymi de Taxone Liber, etc.* In *Corpus Medicorum Latinorum*, vol. 4 (Leipzig, 1927).
2. There is an accessible modern edition of Dioscorides by Robert T. Gunther, ed., *The Greek Herbal of Dioscorides* (1934; London: Hafner, 1968), complete with illustrations from an A.D. 512 Byzantine manuscript and the 1655 text of John Goodyear, who translated his text from the Greek. Latin translations were made soon after Dioscorides completed his work and they circulated and were excerpted throughout Europe. Arber's well-known history, cited earlier, concentrated on printed (not manuscript) herbals. The author briefly traced Dioscorides's work through the Middle Ages and said, "Up to the height of the renaissance period, and later, *De materia medica* was accepted as the almost infallible authority" (Arber, 10). See also John A. Riddle, "The Textual Tradition of Dioscorides in the Latin West," in F. Edward Cranz, ed., *Catalogus Translationum et Commentanorum* IV (1980): 1–143.
3. See for example Pliny the Elder, *Natural History*, trans. H. Rackham, 10 vols. (London: Heinemann, 1938–62).
4. See for example Rudolph E. Siegel, *Galen's System of Physiology and Medicine* (Basel: S. Karger, 1968).
5. Jerry Stannard, "Botanical Data and Late Mediaeval 'Rezeptliteratur' " in Gundolf Keil, *Fachprosa-Studien: Beiträge zur mittelalterlichen Wissenschafts- und Geistesgeschichte* (Berlin: E. Schmidt, 1982), 390. The German word *Rezept* might be translated as recipe, prescription, or remedy. It simply means the directions for preparing a medication out of plants and other (mostly) natural

substances as given in the medieval herbals and other medical texts. *Rezeptliteratur* is a specific term for the literature containing this lore, a genre discussed later in this chapter.

6. For a complete discussion of the title and its author, see Linda Ehrsam Voigts, "The Significance of the Name Apuleius to the Herbarium Apulei," *Bulletin of the History of Medicine* 52 (1978): 214–27, and M. A. D'Aronco and M. L. Cameron, *The Old English Illustrated Pharmacopoeia* (Copenhagen: Rosenkilde and Bagger, 1998), hereafter cited in text as D'Aronco and Cameron.

7. Agnes Arber, cited earlier, discussed the *Herbarium of Pseudo-Apuleius* as one of the first printed herbals and calls it, together with the German *Herbarius* and Latin *Herbarius*, the "doyens among printed herbals" (16), but noted only the *Herbarium* can be traced into antiquity. See especially Augusto Beccaria, *I Codici di Medicina del Periodo Presalernitano (Secoli Ix, X e XI)* (Roma: Edisioni de Storia e Letteratura, 1956), hereafter cited in text as Beccaria. Also refer to D'Aronco and Cameron.

8. See, for example, Peter Brown, *The World of Late Antiquity* (London: Harcourt Brace Jovanovich, 1971) or Norman Cantor, *The Civilization of the Middle Ages* (1963; New York, HarperCollins, 1993).

9. For a discussion of the works that together make up the "enlarged" *Herbarium,* see DeVriend, lv–lxviii. Linda Ehrsam Voigts referred to the work as a "herbal complex" based on the *Herbarium of Pseudo-Apuleius* in "The Old English Herbal in Cotton MS. Vitellius C. III: Studies," (Ph. D. diss. University of Missouri, 1973). Also see John M. Riddle, "Pseudo-Dioscorides' *Ex herbis femininis* and Early Medieval Medical Botany," *Journal of the History of Biology* 14 (1981): 43–81. For the manuscripts of the work in Europe dating earlier than 1100 (before the medical texts from the school of Salerno began to circulate widely), see Beccaria, *I Codici.*

10. Gundolf Keil und Paul Schnitzer, eds., *Das Lorscher Arzneibuch und die Frühmittelalterliche Medizin: Verhandlungen des Medizinhistorischen Symposiums im September 1989 in Lorsch* (Lorsch: Verlag Laurissa, 1991); hereafter cited in text as Keil and Schnitzer. See their introduction for a brief overview of the manuscript, its relationship to the Carolingian reforms, and its place in medical history. The discussions in this book about the *Lorscher Arzneibuch* bear comparing with similar discussions concerning *Bald's Leechbook*; especially provocative is the knowledge that Charlemagne's reforms influenced the Lorsch book strongly, and that King Alfred may have been associated with the compilation of *Bald's Leechbook.* These appear to be similar compilations, although one is in Latin and the other in Old English, but both used a variety of similar sources and only a few of them are in the vernacular.

11. Fundamental to this viewpoint are the writings of Henry E. Sigerist, for example, his *Studien und Texte zur frühmittelalterlichen Rezeptliteratur* (Leipzig: Verlag von J. A. Barth, 1923); hereafter cited in text as Sigerist, *Rezept.* It is noteworthy that Singer often echoed Sigerist, who wrote earlier than he, and seldom cited his works.

12. "Klöster stellten sich als Siedlungsmittelpunkte die medizinische Versorgung, und Klöster sind es gewesen, die als Schaltstellen der Wissenvermit-

tlung über Umfang und Auswahl des medizinischen Traditionsangebotes entschieden." Gundolf Keil, "Möglichkeiten und Grenzen frühmittelalterlicher Medizin" in Keil and Schnitzer, 225.

13. Jerry Stannard, "Marcellus of Bordeaux and the Beginnings of Medieval Materia Medica," *Pharmacy in History* 15, no. 2, (1973): 47; hereafter cited in text as Stannard, "Marcellus." See also Max Niedermann, ed., *Marcellus Über Heilmittel*, 2 vols., 2nd ed. (Berlin: Akademie Verlag, 1968).

14. John M. Riddle, "Theory and Practice in Medieval Medicine," *Viator: Medieval and Renaissance Studies* V (1974): 157–84; hereafter cited in text as Riddle, "Theory."

15. See for example the articles in Jansen-Sieben, ed., *Artes Mechanicae en Europe médiévale/en middeleeuws Europa* (Bruxelles: Archives et Bibliothèques de Belgique, 1989) and in particular Julius Jörimann, "Frühmittelalterliche Rezeptarien," Robert Halleux, "Recettes d'Artisan, Recettes d'Alchimiste," Gundolf Keil, "Die Medizinische Literatur des Mittelalters," and Carmélia Opsomer et Marc Binard, "Materiaux pour une Histoire Quantitative de la Pharmacopée Présalernitaine." Also consult the citations in D'Aronco and Cameron.

16. The School of Salerno has its own extensive body of scholarly literature. Women are known to have studied there, among them Trotula: see Monica Green, "Women's Medical Practice and Health Care in Medieval Europe" in J. M. Bennett, E. A. Clark, J. F. O'Barr, B. A. Vilen, and S. Westphal-Wihl, *Sisters and Workers in the Middle Ages* (Chicago: University of Chicago Press, 1989), 39–78, and *The Trotula* (Philadelphia: University of Pennsylvania Press, 2001). For the medical tradition that began at Salerno, see for example Sigerist or Nancy Siraisi, *Medieval and Early Renaissance Medicine* (Chicago: University of Chicago Press, 1990), and P. O. Kristeller, "The School of Salerno," *Bulletin of the History of Medicine* 17 (1945): 138–94, among a host of other works on this subject.

17. "Nach dem Untergang der antiken Welt brach die trübste Zeit in der Geschichte der medizinischen Wissenschaft an. Galen hatte das medizinische Wissen seiner Zeit in ein gewaltiges System gebracht. Als Schlußstein steht er da, der den Prachtbau der antiken Medizin beschleißt. Mit ihm hört das originelle Schaffen auf, und die folgenden Jahrhunderte gehören den Kompilatoren an. . . . Trüber sah es im römischen Sprachberich aus," Sigerist, *Rezeptliteratur*, iii. The overview of medicine as seen by Sigerist is in his "Vorwort."

18. "Der gemeinsame Grundstock, den die [the Salernitan texts] haben, ist nichts anderes als gerade das Rezeptmaterial des 6./7. Jahrhunderts, zu dem im Laufe der Zeit gelegentlich neue Rezepte hinzukamen oder alte in modernisierter Form."

19. "So glaube ich denn auch, daß wir in den meisten Fällen originale Kompilationen vor uns haben, Sammelungen, die sich der Schreiber für seine klosterärztlichen Bedürfnisse zusammenstellte."

20. Ulrich Stoll, "Das Lorscher Arzneibuch: Ein Überblick über Herkunft, Inhalt und Anspruch des ältesten Arzneibuchs deutscher Provenienz," in Keil and Schnitzer, 73; hereafter cited in text as U. Stoll.

21. Linda Ehrsam Voigts, "Anglo-Saxon Plant Remedies and the Anglo-Saxons," *Isis* 70 (1979): 250–68; hereafter cited in text as Voigts, "Plant Remedies."

22. Gösta Brodin, *Agnus Castus, A Middle English Herbal, Reconstructed from Various Manuscripts* (Uppsala: Lundequistska, 1950). Several manuscripts were used for the study, but the Stockholm MS X 90 was the basic text.

23. For the manuscript tradition of the *Old English Herbarium*, see chapter 4. Also, for example see W. Hofstetter, "Zur lateinischen Quellen des altenglischen Pseudo-Dioskurides," *Anglia* 101 (1983): 315–60.

24. Linda Ehrsam Voigts, "A New Look at a Manuscript Containing the Old English Translation of the Herbarium Apulei," *Manuscripta* 20 (1976): 40–59; "The Significance of the Name Apuleius," and her dissertation, cited earlier.

25. John Harvey, *Medieval Gardens* (London: B. T. Batsford, 1981), 2–3; hereafter cited in text as Harvey. See R. G. Gilligham, "An Edition of Abbot Aelfric's Old English-Latin Glossary with Commentary," (Ph. D. diss. Ohio State University, 1981).

26. "Im Kampf mit den Römern begegnete den Germanen zuerst die antike Medizin, vor allem auch durch die Händler, die den Heeren durch ganz Europa folgten. Auch nach dem Untergang des Römischen Reiches wirkten in den alten Römerstädten die Militärärzte und Chirurgen noch als Zivilärzte und verbreiteten die Kenntnisse der griechisch-römischen Heilkunds im germanischen und gallokeltischen Abendland," Clemens Stoll, "Arznei und Arzneiversorgung in frühmittelalterlichen Klöstern," in Keil and Schnitzer, 153; hereafter cited in text as C. Stoll.

27. "Mit ihrem Wissen und Fertigkeiten und in Verbindung mit dem Handel und den Märkten von Italien bis zur Nordsee verfügten die Klöster auch über eine zeitgemäße Ausstatung und wichtige Vorräte an Lebensmitteln, Medikamenten und Gerätscheften."

28. Miles Hadfield, *Gardens in Britain* (London: Hutchinson, 1960), 17–8. In an interesting note on page 17 of his work, Hadfield said woad, the dye used by the inhabitants of Britain to paint their bodies when they fought Caesar, was native to central and southern Europe, but was cultivated in many other locations already in prehistoric times.

29. Marta Weigle and Peter White, *The Lore of New Mexico* (Albuquerque: University of New Mexico Press, 1988), 328.

30. For historical information, see Peter Hunter Blair, *An Introduction to Anglo-Saxon England* (Cambridge: Cambridge University Press, 1959), chapters 1 and 2; also Peter Brown and Norman F. Cantor, both cited earlier.

31. For the history of New Mexico, see Myra Ellen Jenkins and Albert H. Schroeder, *A Brief History of New Mexico* (Albuquerque: University of New Mexico Press, 1974), 1–32; James T. Burke, *This Miserable Kingdom: The Story of the Spanish Presence in New Mexico and the Southwest from the Beginning until the 18th Century* (Santa Fe, NM: Christo Rey Church, 1973).

32. "In Betracht der Vielfalt der Rezepturen, der Ungenauigkeit der Nomenklatur und der Unsicherheit der Gewichtsumrechnung stellt sich in besonderer Weise die Frage nach den entsprechenden wissenschaftlichen und praktischen Kentnissen der für die Arzneibereitung verantwortlichen Mönche. Die praktischen Fertigkeiten und Erfahrungen konnten nur durch einen längeren

Aufenthalt in einem 'armarium pigmentorum', wie die 'Apotheke' im karolingischen Klosterplan bezeighnet wird, erworben werden. *Diese Kentnisse wurden also auf ganz persönliche Art von Mönch zu Mönch weitergegeben.* Vor allem die irischen Wandermönche, denen die Klöster auf dem Kontinent, zum Beispiel St. Gallen, Lorsch oder Reichenau als Herberge dienten, vermittelten entsprechende Kentnisse aus ihren Heimatklöstern" [emphasis added].

33. Michael Moore, *Los Remedios de la Gente: A Compilation of Traditional New Mexican Herbal Medicines and Their Use* (Santa Fe, NM: 1977), 2; hereafter cited in text as Moore.

34. *Magic and Medicine of Plants,* 9th edition (Pleasantville, NY: Reader's Digest Association, 1997), 27.

35. Heide Grape-Albers, *Spätantike Bilder aus der Welt des Arztes: Medizinische Bilderhandschriften der Spätantike und Ihre Mittelalterliche Überliferund* (Wiesbaden: Guido Pressler Verlag, 1977); hereafter cited in text as Grape-Albers. See Voigts's positive review of Grape-Albers in *Speculum* 57 (1982): 893–95.

36. Minta Collins, *Medieval Herbals: The Illustrative Traditions* (Toronto: University of Toronto Press, 2000).

37. "Neben der fast unübersehbaren Anzahl von Simplicia verfügte die frühmittelalterliche Medizin über eine große Auswahl von Composita. Die Mönche wirkten auch hier sammelnd und ordnend, indem die meist in den überlieferten Schriften verstreut aufgefunden Vorschriften dem gezielten Gebrauch in den Klöstern zugänglich machten. . . . [Antidotaren and Rezepten] waren von den Mönchen des frühen Mittelalters aus den Werken der Antike übernommen und jedoch teilweise dem örtlichen und persönlichen Bedarf angepaßt worden, weshalb kaum eine der anonymen Rezeptsammlungen völlig mit den anderen übereinstimmt."

38. L. S. M. Curtin, *Healing Herbs of the Upper Rio Grande* (Los Angeles: Southwest Museum, 1965), 7; hereafter cited in text as Curtin.

39. "The Foundations of Herbalism" class mentioned above. It was taught one weekend a month for nine months, involving lectures and practical experience with herbal medicine; December 1998 through August 1999. The North American College of Botanical Medicine in Albuquerque, NM, offers a three-year program leading to a bachelor of science degree in herbal medicine and qualifies its graduates to practice as clinical herbologists.

40. L. E. Voigts and Robert P. Hudson, "A drynke þat men callen dwale to make a man to slepe whyle men kerven him: A Surgical Anesthetic from Late Medieval England," in *Health, Disease and Healing in Medieval Culture*, eds. Sheila Campbell, Bert Hall, David Klausner, (New York: St. Martin's Press, 1992), 36; hereafter cited in text as *Dwale.*

41. M. L. Cameron, "Anglo-Saxon Medicine and Magic," *Anglo-Saxon England* 17 (1988): 118; hereafter cited in text as Cameron. See also D'Aronco and Cameron. It is outside the scope of this work to take sides on the current controversy in the United States over whether the U.S. Food and Drug Administration should test and legislate standards for herbal medicines. In other countries, notably Europe, they are a standard part of medical treatment. See

the journal *Fitoterapia* published by Elsevier Science B.V. in which results of tests on ethnobotanical cures are reported from around the world. Information about the journal is available on the Internet at www.elsevier.com/locate/fitote. As of the year 2000, the National Institutes of Health (NIH) in the United States had established a National Center for Complementary and Alternative Medicine (NCCAM) offering grants and research opportunities into healing practices that are outside the mainstream of American medicine, such as the *curanderas*, Native American shamans, and herbologists. The NIH maintains an extensive website and the NCCAM is part of it. See also J. H. Young "Alternative Medicine in the National Institutes of Health," *Bulletin of the History of Medicine* 72 (1998): 279–98.

42. John Mann, *Murder, Magic, and Medicine* (New York: Oxford University Press, 1992), 3; hereafter cited in text as Mann.

43. Bart K. Holland, ed., *Prospecting for Drugs in Ancient and Medieval European Texts: A Scientific Approach* (Amsterdam: Harwood Academic Publishers, 1996), 3.

44. Bart K. Holland, "Prospecting for Drugs in Ancient Texts," *Nature* 369 (30 June 1994): 702.

45. Thurman Hunt, "From Plant Lore to Pharmacy," in Holland 1996, 92.

46. M. Grieve, *A Modern Herbal* (1931; New York: Dover Publications, 1971).

47. Jeanne Rose, *Herbs and Things: Jeanne Rose's Herbal* (New York: Workman, 1973), who dedicated it to "medieval herbalists who felt that to smell green herbs continuously would keep anyone in perfect health." Pages are in parentheses after the quotes.

4

The *Herbarium*

Manuscripts, Illustrations, and the Need for a New Translation

Đeos wyrt, heo hælð wundorliche [This plant cures wonderfully] . . .
—The *Old English Herbarium*

The Anglo-Saxon Manuscripts

The *Old English Herbarium* survives in four manuscripts: Cotton Vitellius C. iii, Hatton 76, and Harley 585, and in Harley 6258B, which is early Middle English. The Early English Text Society Series issued a modern scholarly edition by Jan De Vriend with Latin parallels on the same page as the Old English. For his edition, De Vriend used all of the manuscripts mentioned, manuscripts Cockayne had consulted more than a century earlier. The profusely illustrated Cotton Vitellius C. iii was De Vriend's main text, as it was for Cockayne. As noted earlier, a facsimile edition of the Cotton manuscript was printed in 1998, edited by D'Aronco and Cameron, and in addition, the manuscript is available in microfiche.[1]

Neil Ker's *Catalogue of Manuscripts Containing Anglo-Saxon* discusses the manuscripts in some detail (items 218, 231, 264, and 328), omitting the early Middle English Harley 6258B.[2] The three Old English manuscripts of the *Herbarium of Pseudo-Apuleius* differ only slightly, either because of the translator, because of omissions, or because pages were later misplaced while the manuscript was being rebound. In no instance are the versions widely different. De Vriend's edition completely replaces earlier ones by Hugo Berberich,[3] Aaltje Johanna Geertruida Hilbelink,[4] and Cockayne's hard-to-read transcription. An annotated bibliography appeared in 1992 for the *Old English Herbarium* and the other medical (and magical) Old English texts,[5] and the 1998 facsimile edition by D'Aronco and Cameron not only

updated this bibliography, but included Continental scholars not generally
mentioned in publications on Old English.

De Vriend cited seven manuscripts as parallels to the unknown Latin
original of the *Old English Herbarium;* they range in age from the earliest
extant Latin manuscript of the *Herbarium of Pseudo-Apuleius* to an illustrated manuscript from about A.D. 1250 that shows affinities with earlier versions (De Vriend, xlv–lv). Cockayne had earlier consulted two of them: the
illustrated twelfth-century Harley 5294, and Harley 4986, whose date is
uncertain but is also illustrated (Cockayne 1965, 1:lxxxii–lxxxiii). Apparently no comparison has yet been made of the illustrations in these two manuscripts with the Old English Cotton manuscript. De Vriend did so very
briefly (lv), and for some reason the snakes seem to be an interesting constant in all. The one important tenth-century (or possibly eleventh-century)
Latin manuscript Cockayne obviously did not know about was and is at
Montecassino Monastery in Italy, and it has illustrations that are very similar to the Cotton manuscript; some issues concerning them are discussed
below.

Vitellius C. iii has always been the preferred manuscript to study
because of its illustrations of many of the plants and its generally good condition despite its having been damaged by a fire in 1731 at Ashburnham
House where it was housed. Cockayne called this MS V, a nomenclature De
Vriend retained. Colored drawings of plants and animals throughout the
Herbarium portion distinguish this manuscript from all the others. Hatton 76,
termed MS B by Cockayne and De Vriend, is at the Bodleian Library at
Oxford. The *Herbarium* is on folios 68r through 124r without illustrations,
but with spaces having been left for them that De Vriend notes are nearly the
same size and in the same places as the Cotton (De Vriend, xxii). Harley 585,
MS H for Cockayne and De Vriend, is at the British Museum with the
Herbarium on folios 1r through 101v, and an incomplete table of contents
following on folios 115r through 129v. Also in the British Museum, is Middle English Harley 6258B, the MS O that Cockayne did not use, which displays the *Herbarium* on folios 1r through 44r.

About the dating of the Cotton manuscript, Cockayne cited opinions
saying it dates *as a copy* from about A.D. 1050, but he himself was not as specific, estimating it was not earlier than 1000 or later than 1066 (Cockayne
1965, 1:lxxv). Voigts agreed with Cockayne on a date of about 1050 (see her
dissertation, 23–4); D'Aronco and Cameron favored Ker's dating of the middle of the first half of the eleventh century. All that is certain is that the three
major manuscripts of the *Old English Herbarium* date to the pre-Conquest
eleventh century and MS O to a century later. Charles Singer was alone in
dating the Cotton *Herbarium* to A.D. 950 (Cockayne, 1961, 1:xxi), noting it
was in the Cathedral library of Canterbury, facts Ker considered to be impossible (Ker, 285).

It is still an open question how the three (or four) manuscripts containing the *Old English Herbarium* relate to an earlier lost original. Such a manuscript has not survived but is thought to have existed. In addition to Cockayne's introduction to the *Old English Herbarium*, De Vriend drew, among others, upon a detailed earlier study of *Herbarium Apulei* manuscripts and their tradition by Linda Voigts (Voigts, dissertation). The main focus of Voigts's work was the manuscript tradition to which the Old English versions of the *Herbarium* (especially the Cotton MS) belong, and she discussed the two full-page illustrations at the beginning of Cotton Vitellius C. iii at length in this context. Voigts and De Vriend expressed confidence that there was at least one manuscript in England that served as the prototype to the three eleventh-century Old English works and even possibly to the Montecassino version. De Vriend said, "Although it is more difficult to prove that the original OE version of the Herbarium dates back any further than to the period of the revival of learning in the tenth century, there are some factors which seem to justify the theory that not only the OE MDQ [*Medicina de Quadrupedibus*] but also the OEH came into existence in the period of Northumbrian cultural ascendancy" (De Vriend, xli–xliii, who abbreviated the *Old English Herbarium* as OEH throughout his book). The factors he cited are the supposed existence of both works in Latin in the Northumbrian monasteries in the seventh and eighth centuries and because of the known use of herbs in healing at the time. DeVriend believed certain differences in vocabulary showed that the translations of the *Herbarium of Pseudo-Apuleius* and the *Medicina de Quadrupedibus* might have been made from manuscripts in which the two works had not yet been joined.

D'Aronco presented another view: "On occasion, the [medical] texts evince similarities of form and substance such as to lead us to suppose that at least as early as the late ninth century there had grown up a sort of corpus of remedies in Old English,"[6] she wrote, but found in comparing the remedies in the *Old English Herbarium* with those in the *Leechbooks* and other collections that they were independent translations from Latin sources (yet comparable remedies in the *Lacnunga* match those in the *Herbarium*). She linked the dating of the *Old English Herbarium* to that of the *Leechbook* (the compiler of the *Lacnunga* is known to have used the *Herbarium*, thus postdating it). "It is clear that when the Læceboc was compiled, the translations of the Herbal and the Medicina de Quadrupedibus were not yet available in the form in which they have come down to us. They were only to come into circulation later on and could only subsequently have been consulted for the compilation of other books of remedies" (D'Aronco, Dating).

To reinforce her findings, D'Aronco used considerable evidence from extant glossaries containing the specialized vocabulary of the medical texts, finding that their compilers did not have texts such as the *Old English Herbarium* available at an early time, and demonstrating their relatively late composition. The manuscript traditions to which the *Old English Herbarium* belongs is of background interest to this study because it reinforces the concept of an evolving, fluid corpus of medical texts circulating in Europe and into and around Anglo-Saxon England. However, exactly how particular manuscripts and manuscript stemma relate to each other pertains less here.

The *Herbarium* was a valued work in Anglo-Saxon England, if we can judge by the number of extant manuscripts. As Cockayne remarked in his preface to volume 1, "Its translation into English shows its popularity, and amid the scarcity of old English manuscripts, four copies still exist of this work, and three glossaries show themselves indebted to it" (Cockayne 1965, 1:lxxxviii). D'Aronco went so far as to say that the translation "seems not to have been targeted at the educated (and Latin-speaking) world of the monasteries so much as at a wider public that was not entirely made up of specialists. The Herbal is not presented as a medical treatise and requires no special knowledge of physiology. . . . The Herbal is more similar to a first-aid manual" (D'Aronco, Dating).

To summarize, the *Old English Herbarium* exists in three eleventh-century manuscripts, one of them illustrated, as well as in one from the twelfth century. Two other Old English writings considered to be magico-medical also date from the eleventh century. The manuscripts below contain these vernacular medical texts, which represent the bulk of medical writings known to survive from Anglo-Saxon and very early Anglo-Norman England (see Ker 264):

Cotton Vitellius C. iii (British Library) includes the illustrated *Old English Herbarium,* which is the text used for Cockayne 1961 and 1965, vol. 1, and is called MS V by Cockayne and DeVriend (listed as Ker 218).

Hatton 76 (Bodleian Library) has the *Old English Herbarium* with spaces left for illustrations but none in place; it is called MS B in Cockayne and De Vriend, who used it for comparison with V (listed as Ker 328).

Harley 585 (British Library) has the *Old English Herbarium,* called MS H in Cockayne and De Vriend, and both used it for comparison with MS V. This manuscript also contains the collection of recipes and charms known as the *Lacnunga,* printed in Cockayne's volume 3, and also the *Lorica* of Gildas in Latin with Old English glosses. De Vriend noted there are a few marginal sketches in the *Herbarium* section, mainly of serpents (listed as Ker 231).

Harley 6258B is the twelfth-century manuscript that contains the *Old English Herbarium,* and was called MS O by Cockayne and De Vriend. De Vriend pointed out that its organization differs from all the others (not listed in Ker).

Royal 12 D. xvii (British Museum) contains medical recipes, charms, and the Old English work that Cockayne called *Bald's Leechbook,* which is in Cockayne's volume 2. (See Marilyn Deegan, "A Critical

Edition of MS. B.L. Royal 12. D. XVII: Bald's 'Leechbook' Vols. 1
and 2," (Ph. D. diss., University of Manchester, 1988). This work, the
Lacnunga, and the *Old English Herbarium* represent the major surviving medical texts from Anglo-Saxon England.

The Illustrations in the Cotton *Old English Herbarium*

Of all the manuscripts containing the *Old English Herbarium*, Cotton Vitellius C. iii is unique because of its illustrations. The subject of several specialized studies, the illustrations are of secondary interest here. Following the
argument presented in chapter 3, from the standpoint of their use to the
reader, the plant drawings should be considered aids to memory, schematics
to assist someone who knew the plants fresh or dried. The three title pages of
human figures at the beginning of the manuscript helped establish the authority of the work for the medieval reader as coming from ancient and accepted
sources, but even without them, the *Herbarium* was so very well known, such
illustrations were unnecessary. The authorities simply added to the value and
usefulness of this codex. That all the illustrations can be linked to Continental sources bolsters the thesis advanced earlier that Anglo-Saxon medicine
can be closely linked to a pan-European tradition.

The illustrations in the Cotton manuscript consist of: (1) three title pages
on 11v, 19r, and 19v; (2) plant illustrations that are placed near the beginning
of every entry in the body of the *Herbarium* and exist for every plant but the
last one; (3) snakes, spiders, and scorpions appearing near the remedies in the
Herbarium that would be made to cure the poison from their bite; and (4)
animals that were used in preparing the remedies in the *Medicina de Quadrupedibus,* a work not covered here.

The three illuminated title pages have been the subject of considerable
discussion, in fact more so than the numerous drawings of plants, animals,
and snakes that accompany the remedy portion of the work. On 19r is a
framed image with a large central figure holding plants in his hands, a centaur to his left, and a figure in classical robes to his right; below the frame are
the names Escolapius, Plato, Centaurus. Above and below the human figures
are animals and snakes. On 19v is the title of the work—*Herbarium Apulei
Platonici Quod Acceptit Ab Escolapio et Alchirone Centauro Magis<t>ro
Achillis*—encircled in a frame. Voigts, who has studied the illustrations in
this manuscript extensively, interpreted these folios together as being author
portraits, examples of a standard type of illustration present in herbals from
classical times through the Middle Ages.

> This author portrait is found between the table of contents and the first
> chapter of the herbal; it depicts the source of and the authority for the rem-
> edy book. Portrayed in this miniature are Aesculapius, Chiron, and, in the

center, the putative author of the herbal, Apuleius Platonicus, often desig-
nated in herbals as Plato or Plato Apoliensis.[7]

Voigts suggested the title on the reverse explained that the Plato/Apuleius
figure was receiving the book from the two patrons of medicine.

D'Aronco, who wrote the section on codicology and paleography for the
facsimile edition already cited, interpreted the drawing slightly differently.
She found that the scene illustrates the contents of the manuscript (the herbal
portion by the plants in Plato's hands and the *Medicina de Quadrupedibus* by
the animals in the background). She suggested that Aesculapius and Chiron's
handing the herbal to the mortal author Plato was "a symbolic act, represent-
ing the passage of medical knowledge from the gods to mortals, while at the
same time attributing the paternity of the work to an undisputed authority
who confers on it legitimacy and status" (D'Aronco and Cameron, 26). In the
opinion of both Voigts and D'Aronco, these title page illustrations can be
traced in content and style to late classical types.

Less conclusive are their discussions about the illustration on folio 11v,
which begins the *Herbarium* portion of the Cotton manuscript, coming
before the table of contents. Here is found a large central figure who is standing on what appears to be a lion, holding a spear in his right hand and a book
in his left. The lion appears to be biting the spear. To his right is a tonsured
figure holding out a book to him, and at the bottom left is a Roman soldier.
Cockayne thought that this was a dedicatory page to begin the manuscript,
and that one of the figures "depicts the church dignitary for whom the work
was copied, one a tonsured priest presenting a volume, and one is soldier
with a roman air" (Cockayne 1965, 1:lxxvii). However, no inscription is
present to aid in identifying any of the figures.

Voigts said that a dedication page such as this one, like the author/
portrait page on 19r, was a classical genre, but she linked it in style to the
monastery of Saint-Bertin in French Flanders (Voigts, "New Look," 48–50).
Further, she identified the central figure with Anglo-Saxon tomb sculpture,
concluding that the codex was dedicated to a bishop or abbot-saint "of particular importance to the house which produced or commissioned the work"
(Voigts, "New Look," 54). Here, she again pointed to northern France for
similar depictions, but conceded that the identity of the figure might never be
known. About the other two figures, Voigts said only that one was a monk,
the other a "non-royal lay donor, a phenomenon rare in Anglo-Saxon manuscripts," and observed generally about the dedication page that it was "highly
irregular among Anglo-Saxon dedication pages" (Voigts, "New Look," 55).

D'Aronco, on the other hand, questioned whether this page really
depicts a dedication scene, arguing that it "ought to be viewed as a composition with a semantic structure of its own that can be read only in the context
of the work it is intended to illustrate, that is within the traditional iconogra-

phy of herbals" (D'Aronco and Cameron, 29). Her conclusion was that this page "could be the result of the conflation of single author-portraits modernized according to contemporary canons" (D'Aronco and Cameron, 30). She suggested that the central figure depicts the author of the text, Aesculapius or Apollo/Apuleius, and that the other two figures bring up to date a discussion scene of two figures associated with healing, Antonius Musa and Marcus Agrippa (who are transformed respectively into a monk and a Roman soldier holding a scroll).

Studies of the plant illustrations have also tended to focus on who copied which model, thus helping establish manuscript stemma. Attention is generally called only to those few illustrations that clearly do not depict the plant called out in the text, yet it is remarkable how closely many illustrations capture the essential appearance of the plants, albeit in almost cartoon fashion. They look remarkably similar to pressed plants, such as are found in modern botanical herbariums. The most up-to-date study for the illustrations in all the known manuscripts of the Pseudo-Apuleius herbal is the work by Grape-Albers, which traces the history of illustrated Pseudo-Apuleius manuscripts from late-classical times through the Middle Ages.[8] She used the illustrations to help establish that the manuscript families proposed long ago by Howald and Sigerist for the *Herbarium of Pseudo-Apuleius* were essentially correct, and also argued that in every instance, the texts (even when excerpted) and their plant illustrations remained together through the centuries the manuscripts of this work circulated and were recopied (Grape-Albers, 13–21 and 164–6; D'Aronco and Cameron, 31–8, base their discussion on this study). Outside the scope of the present study, but an interesting question, is the possible relationship of the Cotton manuscript to another at Montecassino from about the same period whose illustrations appear remarkably similar to it. Grape-Albers put them in the same family. In her dissertation, Voigts did not agree, finding that the Old English may have been the source for the Italian manuscript (Voigts, diss., 56 ff.). (The many illustrated versions of the *Herbarium* are also discussed in Minta Collins's work, cited earlier.)

The snake and scorpion paintings in the manuscript are an interesting side issue. Cockayne believed these illustrations, which are prominently placed throughout the *Herbarium*, were entirely fanciful, and it must be said they have received little attention, the plants being the main interest. However, in a study connecting with the *Herbarium of Pseudo-Apuleius* the snakes that are called out by name in Wolfram's *Parzifal*, Arthur Gross showed that from an early time remedies for snakebite, for wounds caused by weapons poisoned with snake venom, and drawings of snakes were an important part of the *Herbarium* and remained a constant part of its transmission.[9] It is no doubt that the snakes, spiders, and scorpions were important to this work: remedies for bites from such creatures outnumber those for any other single complaint, numbering about forty-eight instances. In terms of their frequency mentioned, the next most common conditions addressed are stomach and abdominal pain and swelling (forty-three) and various kinds of wounds and sores (forty-five), which are each usually described with considerable detail so the healer can decide whether the remedy offered is appropriate to use on that type sore. Although no real conclusions can drawn from the frequency of conditions cited, they are informative. Numbering far fewer than the three areas mentioned, but fairly frequently called out are eye conditions (twenty-four), constipation and diarrhea (ten each), inability to urinate (twenty), bladder stones and pain (fifteen), fever (seventeen), headache (twenty), worms around the anus (ten), aching joints (eleven), pain in the spleen (thirteen), swellings (eighteen), gout (fifteen), antidotes to poison (ten), and dropsy (eight). Conditions specific to women are mentioned in sixteen instances, and some of the remedies may have been intended to produce abortions (they are noted in the text) though they do not say so specifically.

The snakes and scorpions certainly cannot be missed when looking through the manuscript pages; they are lively and stand out, perhaps clearly marking a cure for a poisonous bite if someone needed to find it in a hurry. D'Aronco noted that the reptiles and insects can in some instances be recognized.

> Snakes and serpents in Vitellius C. iii are depicted in such lavish detail that the species portrayed is sometimes recognizable, as, for example, the snake on fol. 32v, col. 2, whose head is adorned with horns and wattles. This is clearly *Cerastes cerastes* (= *C. Cornutus*), the sand viper, and we note a similar care for detail in the snake on fol. 49r, col. 1, in which we can recognize a water snake (*chersydros*). (D'Aronco and Cameron, 41)

The illustrations of plants, animals, reptiles, and snakes served to make a book of remedies such as the *Old English Herbarium* and its parent, the *Herbarium of Pseudo-Apuleius*, even more useful. But even without illustrations, the work was popular and used. The title pages may have had meaning to the medieval user of these manuscripts that is not entirely clear to us, but they were obviously of some importance because of their continuation in use from late classical times into the Renaissance.

Need for a New Translation: Misconceptions Created by Cockayne

The reader who consults only Cockayne's English translation of Anglo-Saxon medical works is easily misled about (1) the intended use for the herbal—the remedies appear to be only for men, (2) about the seeming absence of complaints specific to women—Cockayne disguised some of them in Latin or Greek, and (3) about the seriousness of the text—Cockayne's style casts doubts immediately on the nature of the remedies.

Cockayne chose to translate most of the remedies in the following manner: "If a mans head be broken. . . . In case a mans inwards be too costive. . . . In case blood gush up through a mans mouth. . . . In case a carbuncle is going to settle on a man" (Cockayne 1965, 1:3; note that he used "mans" for man's). The Old English word Cockayne was translating is the indefinite *man,* which meant "one," just like the modern German word *man.* Even in the English of Cockayne's day, "a man" was a gender-specific term, and there was no linguistic reason to use it, particularly in such frequent formulas as *Wiþ þæt man . . . sy,* which Cockayne invariably translated as "In case a man be . . ." Translating the Anglo-Saxon word *man* as "a person" or "one" is closer to its meaning in the original. The Latin manuscripts on which most of the texts were based used a passive construction, hence implying no gender for the remedy. The following excerpts from the first entry in the *Herbarium* concerning uses for betony illustrate the subtle shift that occurred in translation from Latin to Anglo-Saxon to Cockayne (and to Grattan-Singer as well).

Latin text: *Ad alvum concitandum. . . . ad sanguinem qui per os reiciunt et purulentum. . . . ad carbunculos* (De Vriend 1984, 33–5). Anglo-Saxon text: *Gif mannes innod to faest sy. . . . wiþ þe men blod up welle. . . . Gif man wylle spring on gisittan* (Cockayne 1965, 1:2, and in DeVriend 1984, 33 and 35). Cockayne's translation: In case a mans inwards be too costive. . . . in case blood gush up through a mans mouth. . . . in case a pustule is going to settle on a man. (Cockayne 1965, 1:3)

A complementary, but perhaps understandable, bias in Cockayne in view of his profession and the time in which he lived, was his habit of sometimes lapsing into Latin and Greek instead of straightforward English when he encountered a remedy dealing with female functions. However Victorian this delicate avoidance might be, it is misleading for a reader who cannot consult the Latin or Anglo-Saxon originals and is depending on Cockayne for information. Such a reader might be left with the impression that the Anglo-Saxons did not deal in a straightforward manner with "delicate" subjects, when they did. For example, an Anglo-Saxon passage begins, *"Wið wifes flewsan genim ðas yclan wyrte on mortere wel gepunude . . ."* and without explanation, in the middle of his translation into modern English, Cockayne wrote, *"Ad mulieris fluxus, herbam hanc in mortario tusam, ita ut omnino lenta fiat . . ."* (Cockayne 1965, 1:312–13).

However, the most serious misconception Cockayne's translation creates is that medieval medicine was frivolous. By using antiquated and contorted turns of phrase in translating the Old English, Cockayne may have sought to give a flavor of the old language, but, as discussed in chapter 2, it came across as ridiculous even in the nineteenth century. Language style very much affects how information is received. "Worts, wambs, ill runnings of the inwards, head breaches, swart roots, and a sun that upgoeth" (all taken from Cockayne's *Leechdoms*) are not terms that connote serious medicine, and the prefaces Cockayne supplied to each of the three volumes of the *Leechdoms* tend to reinforce a negative attitude toward Anglo-Saxon and medieval medicine, as mentioned earlier.

In the nearly 150 years since Cockayne's translation was published, attitudes about many aspects of language and ancient medicine have changed, and there is a need for an updated version of the translated text and new material about the medicine. The philosophy behind the present translation is that this was a text used to transmit information on the healing properties of plants and how to administer them. The *Old English Herbarium* is one of several key texts in understanding late classical and medieval medicine in Western Europe, and a modern translation will allow it to be used by a wider audience. Notwithstanding the need to update Cockayne's translations and, as indicated earlier, the prefaces, these remarks are not intended to diminish his contribution to scholarship; he in fact transcribed, translated, and thus made available nearly all the known Anglo-Saxon medical texts. Any discussion of Anglo-Saxon medicine or magic will necessarily and always begin with Cockayne.

In the three-volume *Leechdoms,* Cockayne's transcriptions of the Old English manuscripts are printed on pages that face his translations so the reader can compare them easily. The typeface for the transcriptions must have been designed specifically for the Rolls Series editions of Anglo-Saxon; it replicated the form of the manuscript letters. It is unfortunate that none of the correspondence between Cockayne and his printer survived, because a good amount of effort obviously went into designing the typeface and ensuring the printer could correctly copy Cockayne's handwritten transcriptions. Cockayne referred to his work as a "facsimile" in volume 1 of the *Leechdoms* (lxxv), and he noted that he did not normalize the Anglo-Saxon, deferring to the original manuscripts for the following reason:

> The text has been printed in the form, as regards the shape of the characters, which they take in the original MSS. Besides the objection to printing in the character of our own day, which arises in the heart of every man who dislikes to dress up antiquity in modern clothes, there is one which is not sentimental at all; by a change in levelling we lose all the chronological characteristics of a manuscript arising from the form of the letters. (Cockayne 1965, 1:xc)

In this same preface, Cockayne discussed what he considered to be the dangerous consequences of establishing a standard version of Old English and normalizing an edition of a text to that standard. His main reason, as he stated above, was that the forms of the letters give a clue as to the age of the manuscript, and he thought it important to preserve in print the form of the letters in the manuscript he was using. Known always as an extremely exact and careful scholar, as outlined in chapters 1 and 2, Cockayne established Cotton Vitellius C iii as his main text for the *Herbarium* in his preface. In the printed version, he referred to variant readings in other manuscripts at the bottom of each page. In spot checks with De Vriend's edition and with D'Aronco and Cameron, it must be said Cockayne's transcriptions are very exact.

In keeping with his desire to provide a facsimile, rather than an edition, of the *Old English Herbarium*, Cockayne did not punctuate the Anglo-Saxon text, as most editors are inclined to do, De Vriend included. Imitating the original, Cockayne provided capital letters at the beginning of paragraphs and then printed the remainder of the paragraph without added punctuation. His editorial decisions were limited to deciphering letters that were nearly impossible to distinguish clearly and in separation of some words that were run together in the manuscript. The points Cockayne raised about editing and printing Anglo-Saxon works are still valid. He was quite concerned about the effect an editor has on the interpretation and reception of a given work. Cockayne's remarks are in the preface to volume 1 of the *Leechdoms* (Cockayne 1965, 1:xc–cv) and outline his philosophy of editing Old English texts.

Sources Used in the Present Translation

This translation of the *Old English Herbarium* was based primarily on De Vriend's 1984 edition of the work supplemented by D'Aronco and Cameron's facsimile. Cockayne's translation of it was both a source and in some instances a hurdle to overcome. Note is made where the present translation differs appreciably from Cockayne's, but not everything in his translation was addressed, particularly when it was unclear what it adds to our understanding of the original. For example, Cockayne's use of Greek names, Greek spellings, and Greek letters for some of the plants (and sometimes the conditions) was not noted or retained here, that being considered a separate object of study (see Cockayne 1961 or 1965 for his use of Greek in the *Herbarium* translation). In the original manuscripts, no distinction was made in the way Latin and Greek words were written. Cockayne seemed to be pointing out to us that he knew which plant names were Greek and, as a good philologist of his day, wanted to be correct and wrote them using Greek letters, correcting the form in the original at times, even the name. His sources for the Greek are not known. However, use of synonyms in several languages for plant names became a traditional part of medieval herbals and it is misleading to call attention to any one form by using Greek letters. Granted, it is misleading (but required) here to bow to current convention and put the Latin and Greek forms in italics, as well. We do not know the preferred name for a plant in Anglo-Saxon times; it may well have been one of the classical names, as is the case today for people who use botanical names easily when talking about plants.

References used for Old English plant names were Cockayne, De Vriend's edition of the *Old English Herbarium, The Old English Illustrated Pharmacopoeia* by D'Aronco and Cameron, Peter Bierbaumer's *Der botanische Wortschatz des Altenglishen* (1975) and Tony Hunt's *Plant Names of Medieval England* (1989).[10] It should be noted that the work of D'Aronco and Cameron includes all of the sources mentioned here in discussing plant identification as well as very recent work being published on the subject; as of 1999, it was the most complete published study of the *Old English Herbarium*. Because D'Aronco and Cameron's was the only work that used all earlier sources to identify the plants in the *Herbarium*, theirs are the plant names used in the present translation.

With regard to Cockayne's identification of plants, he gives no sources for his botanical knowledge. Immediately preceding his glossary in volume 3 of the *Leechdoms*, he stated that his work "relies almost entirely upon original author-ities; upon a collation of the manuscript ancient extant glossaries with their printed editions, which have been falsified by ignorant conjectures; and upon a careful examination of many Saxon volumes never yet published. No reliance has been placed on modern productions, in the way of dictionaries; they will be found full of errors" (Cockayne 1965, 3:363). The final statement recalls his 1864 attack on Bosworth's *Anglo-Saxon Dictionary*, and Cockayne here foot-noted his own publication with reference to the slur on modern dictionaries: *The Shrine* of 1864. (As noted earlier, it is extremely difficult to identify Cockayne's sources from the notes he provided in the *Leechdoms* and in other works.)

Supplemental information on herbs and plants came from Grieve's *A Modern Herbal, Culpepper's Herbal, The Greek Herbal of Dioscorides*, (see bibliography for complete citations),[11] Malcolm Stuart, *Encyclopedia of Herbs and Herbalism,* and from the several classes and workshops previ-ously mentioned in the text.

Abbreviations for sources frequently cited in the footnotes are as follows:

C: Cockayne's translation of the *Old English Herbarium*
BT: Bosworth-Toller's *Anglo-Saxon Dictionary*
D'A: D'Aronco and Cameron, *The Old English Illustrated Pharma-copoeia*
DeV: De Vriend *Old English Herbarium*
DOE: *Dictionary of Old English*
Other works are cited by the author's last name

Where the current translation differs appreciably from Cockayne's, the Old English term in question is cited in a note, then Cockayne's translation is given as C = ⸺.

Today, the units of measure in the *Herbarium* are regarded generally with despair, either because their meaning is not known with any exactitude, as in the case of *sester* (a jar or pitcher), or because the weight or size of something such as a penny's weight or a spoonful is also not clear to us. The necessity of not relying entirely on what is written in this work and works like it cannot be overemphasized—they will never be completely understood merely by reading the medical treatise. Reading the work must be coupled some familiarity with medicinal plants and their uses, so that one can decide how much of the directions to follow explicitly and how much to alter—the *Old English Herbarium* and works like it should be used as a guidebook and a reference, not as a manual on how to prescribe and make herbal remedies. De Vriend discussed modern equivalents of Anglo-Saxon and Roman weights and measures on pages lxxxi–lxxxiv, and these equivalents were generally used to convert the measures given in the *Herbarium* into modern terms.

Notes on the Translation

This is not a literal translation in the sense that Cockayne's is. His work is available to those who want to read a more-or-less word-for-word rendition of the Anglo-Saxon. No attempt was made to mimic the Old English word order, and many filler words (then, and) were omitted, as was some of the repetition (for example, "that same plant"). By not providing a literal translation, some interesting turns of phrase present in Old English were unfortunately lost. Two major considerations had to be weighed: (1) faithfulness to the Old English and (2) transmitting information accurately to modern readers of English (not necessarily to those who can read Latin or Anglo-Saxon). The most literal translation of a term or phrase was used as far as possible. But where that literal meaning would confuse a modern reader, the closest approximation to the Old English was chosen when it had a clear meaning in modern English.

Verbs such as *cnucian* (*cnocian*), "to pound," posed a challenge, because plants can be bruised, mashed, crushed, pulverized, or chopped, all with the same general action as being pounded, and indeed, the Anglo-Saxons, like the classical healers, used a mortar and pestle to pound and crush their medicinal plants—today's herbologists may use a blender! The most frequent verb in the original for a means to pulverize fresh and dried plants is *cnucian* (to pound). It has been retained because (1) that is what is in the text and (2) it can be understood by anyone familiar with herbal preparations as a general instruction to break up the plant somehow so that its essential oils and juices will work more readily in the preparation. Another challenge was the verb *wyllan* (literally, to boil). At hands-on workshops on preparation of medicinal herbal remedies, the caution was generally given never to boil (truly boil hard) herbs; instead, they are simmered or cooked just below the boiling point (one *curandera* said the water should be "smiling"). To reflect accurately both the verb and customary practice, here, *wyllan* was translated as "to gently boil." *Seoðan* (to seethe or simmer) could have meant either simmer or actually to seethe (infuse)—in reality, both produce nearly the same result—and in observing preparations being made, the medieval practitioner would have learned the subtle difference between "simmer" and "seethe," which were used nearly interchangeably here.

"Worms about the navel" (*nafolan*) is a condition mentioned several times, usually in the context of their being intestinal worms, thus not worms associated with a skin condition. Intestinal worms would have often manifested themselves at the anus, and a medical consultant said that the anus or a knot of skin like it—as well as the navel—are often referred to today as an umbilicum. Indeed, *Merriam-Webster's Medical Dictionary* defines an umbilication as a depression resembling an umbilicus. *Umbilicus* is the term used in the hypothetical Latin original of the *Old English Herbarium* for where these worms appear, and the worms are called *lumbrici,* sometimes with *et tinae* added. Marcellus of Bordeaux devoted chapter 28 to curing various kinds of intestinal worms (*lumbrici et tinae*) using similar remedies as the *Herbarium.*[12] Most involve drinking an herb or mixture of herbs to kill and expel the worms and/or applying or inserting the herbs (in)to the anus. It seems likely that the worms referred to here were intestinal worms that appeared at the anus (a fairly common condition) rather than navel worms, a condition largely unheard of. For this reason, the translation here for *nafolan* is anus when referring to the condition of worms about the *nafolan.*

By necessity, a translation is an interpretation, not just of the words but of the work itself. The interpretation guiding this work is that the *Herbarium* was not intended to be a step-by-step manual in preparing drugs and treating people. Instead, the *Herbarium* and medieval medical works like it were notes for preparations, notes to help one decide what to prescribe for a condition, as are contemporary works on medicinal plants.

Most of the remedies follow a formula of the pattern (1) for this condition, (2) take the plant, (3) prepare it in a certain manner, (4) administer it, (5) this is the result you can expect. Not all parts of the formula are always present, and the actions are generally not explained. For example how one "collects" (picks, harvests, digs up, cuts, etc.) the plant, details on the preparation other than seethe or mix, and how to administer it other than "put it on" are sometimes omitted. And often, the object of the action is missing entirely, and one is directed to seethe the plant in water and give to drink, or, to treat a wound, to pound a plant with fat and put it on. Such terse instructions have usually been retained in this translation, the rationale being that the object is clearly understood from the context and that many remedy books written even today employ such shorthand. Common is the instruction, for example, to pound a plant in wine and give to drink, shorthand for pound the plant until it is pulverized, put it into a certain amount of wine, let it seep in the wine for some length of time (depending on the plant and how long it takes for its essential oils to infuse into the liquid), perhaps strain the liquid, and then give it to the patient to drink. The same is true for the frequent instruction: Pound the plant in grease and put it on. Here again, the plant would be pulverized fresh or dry, mixed with the grease, the salve would be allowed to rest for some time, and then the salve put on the patient's wound. Herbal medicine has always relied on apprenticeship (much as modern medicine does for the *practicum* of medicine), and it is clear that this text was written for someone who knew how to use its abbreviated instructions. What is found here was not for a "student leech," a term coined by Olds, but instead was wisdom transmitted from one healer to another. Informed users would have been able to supply missing information from their own store of practical knowledge. Just as in cooking, the recipes one follows benefit from seeing and experiencing what is actually meant by simmer, cook, boil gently, a rolling boil, cook just below the boiling point, and so forth.

The Latin original was equally terse and expressed in the passive voice, and the translation into Old English presented an entirely different style from the original, but it followed fairly closely what was there and merely adapted it to the foreign idiom. In a few of the remedies, there is a personal note that someone (we or I) attested to how well it worked, but that is rare. And, yes, there were mistakes in translation and omissions in going from the Latin to Old English—nevertheless, this text existed as we see it and it was used despite its flaws. This translation, if it meets its purpose, will help transmit information to anyone interested in the topic of medieval medicine or the history of use of medicinal plants; in addition, it will supply a better understanding of medical and botanical references in literary and historical texts.[13] It is definitely not intended to demonstrate the quaintness of medieval medicine—far from it. Cockayne's three volumes do that extremely well. The main intent is to provide an accurate and useful version of the *Old English Herbarium* as a witness of an unbroken tradition of healing from before this millennium, through it, and on to the next.

As to the problem of being able to identify correctly the 185 plants in the *Herbarium*, a small number may never be identified to everyone's satisfaction. However, it is remarkable that a very large number of them have been identified with certainty, given the huge geographic area and the great span of time involved in the long life of this work. Moreover, in practice, healers have always sought varieties of plants to help the ill wherever they might be living. This text was used in medieval Europe over many centuries from Italy to England and Scandinavia. Using it would have surely entailed many substitutions of varieties of plants in the same family, and this would have affected how the text was transmitted. Merely because *we* cannot identify plants based on the illustrations and descriptions given in this and other manuscripts does not necessarily mean that the writers and illustrators did not know what they were doing. Rather, we need to bring new eyes and new sensibilities to the texts. Despite mistranslations, mistakes, and omissions in the *Old English Herbarium*, it is important to remember that at least four copies existed at nearly the same time in Anglo-Saxon England, and *these are what were used.*

Contents for the Herbarium: The Old English original has an unnumbered contents list; however, to facilitate comparison with Cockayne and De Vriend, their numbered lists have been retained, albeit using arabic rather than the cumbersome roman numerals that they employed. The numbering follows De Vriend, not Cockayne, although there is scant difference between them. The original *Old English Herbarium* did not number anything; this was Cockayne's addition. In the translated contents list, the first plant name appears just as it does in the original, followed by a translation of the Old English term if there was one. Often, no Old English plant name was provided.

The remedies in the Herbarium: In the translation of the *Herbarium*'s remedies, following the list of contents, each section begins with the customary modern English name followed by its official botanical name in parentheses, then the Latin or Greek name as found in the Old English work, and finally the Old English plant name if one was in the manuscript. The remedies are given subsection numbers which did not exist in the original.

The Cotton manuscript is laid out so that there are two columns of text on each page. Following the contents list, a large illustration begins each section of the *Herbarium*, identifying the plant that is named and featured in the remedies. The Old English name of the plant, if such existed, is an integral part of the illustration. If there was no Old English name for the plant, the Latin name was used. Sometimes, but rarely, no name was inserted. Only the final entry has no illustrated section heading.

Plant names: As noted, the plant names agree with those in D'Aronco and Cameron.

The snakes: A drawing of a snake appears in the translation where a snake appears in Cotton Vitellius C. iii, and a scorpion is used to mark where the original had an insect or scorpion. Many of the remedies appear to be for venomous bites generally, whether from a snake, spider, or other creature.

Notes

1. Cotton Vitellius C. iii is in volume 1 of the *Anglo-Saxon Manuscripts in Microfiche Facsimile* (Binghamton, NY: Medieval & Renaissance Texts & Studies, 1994).
2. Neil R. Ker, *Catalogue of Manuscripts Containing Anglo-Saxon* (Oxford: Clarendon Press, 1957); hereafter cited in text as Ker.

3. Hugo Berberich, ed., *Das Herbarium Apulei nach einer früh-mittelenglischen Fassung* (1901; Amsterdam: Swets und Zeitlinger NV Nachgedruckt, 1966). This is Harley 6258B, the MS O. Cockayne did not use. Berberich's study contains twelve pages about the MS and the script, 'Lautlehre' on pages 14–30, grammar on pages 33–6, and the text makes up pages 65–138. The edition contains no commentary or glossary.

4. Aaltje Johanna Geertruida Hilbelink, *Cotton MS Vitellius C. iii of the Herbarium Apulei* (Amsterdam: NV Swets und Zeitlanger, 1930). This dissertation has a very general two-page introduction and only cites Cockayne. After the edited text is a short study of forms by grammatical class.

5. Stephanie Hollis and Michael Wright, *Old English Prose of Secular Learning* (Cambridge: D. S. Brewer, 1992).

6. M. A. D'Aronco, "The Old English Herbal: A Proposed Dating for the Translation," unpublished English translation (quoted with permission of the author) of "L'erbario anglosassone, un'ipotesi sulla data della traduzione," *Romanobarbarica* 13 (1995, pub. 1996), 325–365; hereafter cited in text as D'Aronco, Dating.

7. Linda Ehrsam Voigts, "A New Look at the Manuscript Containing the Old English Translation of the *Herbarium Apulei*," *Manuscripta* 20 (1976): 42; hereafter cited in text as Voigts, "New Look"). See also her article "The Significance of the Name Apuleius to the *Herbarium Apulei*," *Bulletin of the History of Medicine* 52 (1978): 214–27; hereafter cited in text as Voigts, Apuleius.

8. Grape-Albers has issued a new facsimile of Vienna 93, the focus of her earlier study; see her *Medicina Antiqua: Codex Vindobonensis 93* (London: Harvey Miller, 1999), with an introduction by Peter Murray Jones. See also Minta Collins's *Medieval Herbals* for a discussion of the illustrative traditions in Greek, Arabic, and Latin herbals through the fifteenth century. Of related interest is Peter Murray Jones, *Medieval Medicine in Illuminated Manuscripts* (London: British Library, 1998).

9. Arthur Gross, "Wolframs Schlangenliste (*Parzifal* 481) und Pseudo-Apuleius," in *Licht der Natur: Medizin in Fachliteratur und Dichtung*, eds. J. Domes, W. Gerabek, B. Haage, C. Weißer, und V. Zimmermann (Göppingen: Kümmerle Verlag, 1994), 128–48. Gross based some of his arguments on Grape-Albers.

10. For those primarily interested in the linguistic aspects of the vocabulary in this and other medical writings in Old English (word formation and so forth), see Hans Sauer's articles "Towards a Linguistic Description and Classification of the Old English Plant Names," in *Words, Texts and Manuscripts: Studies in Anglo-Saxon Culture Presented to Helmut Gneuss*, ed. M. Korhammer et al. (Cambridge: D. S. Brewer, 1992), 381–408; "On the Analysis and Structure of Old and Middle English Plant Names," in *The History of English*, No. 3, 1997, 133–61; and "English Plant Names in the Thirteenth Century: The Trilingual Harley Vocabulary," *Middle English Miscellany*, ed. Jacek Fisiak (Posnan: Motivex, 1996), 135–55. See also M. A. D'Aronco, "The Botanical Lexicon of the Old English Herbarium," *Anglo-Saxon England* 17 (1988): 15–33; J. M. Bately, "Old English Prose Before and During the Reign of Alfred," *Anglo-Saxon England* 17 (1988): 93–138.

11. Concerning identification of plants in medieval texts, D'Aronco and Cameron, and Tony Hunt, *Plant Names of Medieval England* (Cambridge: D. S. Brewer, 1989) use J. André, *Lexique des termes de botanique en latin* (Paris: Klincksieck, 1956), which De Vriend (1984) does not cite, though it was available when his edition was made. In addition, D'Aronco and Cameron use G. Maggiulli and M.F. Buffa Giolito, *L'altro Apuleio. Problemi aperti per una nuova edizione dell'Herbarius* (Naples, 1996) cited as "*Nomenclatura della piante.*" All use Bierbaumer (1975–1979, vols. 1–3). In addition, an Anglo-Saxon Plant Name Survey (APSN) now exists at the University of Glasgow, a research project of the Institute for the Historical Study of Language, and its first symposium was held in April of 2000. Complete information about the ASPN is available on the Internet at http://www2.arts.gla.ac.uk/EngLang/ihsl/projects/ASPNS/info.htm.

12. Marcellus of Bordeaux, *Marcellus Über Heilmittel*, vol. 2, ed. Max Nidermann (Berlin: Akademie Verlag, 1968), 486–93.

13. See William T. Stearn, *Botanical Latin* (Portand, OR: Timber Press, 1998) for a complete discussion of the history, grammar, syntax, terminology, and vocabulary of botanical Latin.

5

A New Translation of the
Old English Herbarium

***Herbarium:* Contents**

The chapters of the book of medicine begin:

21. For abdominal pain or swelling
22. For drinking poison
23. For snakebite
24. For snakebite
25. For bite of a mad dog
26. For a sore throat or part of the neck
27. For sore loins or an ache in the thighs
28. For high fever
29. For gout

2. The *arniglosa* plant, which is **common plantain**
   1. For headache
   2. For stomach pain
   3. For abdominal pain
   4. Again, for a swollen stomach
   5. For anal bleeding
   6. For wounds
   7. To soften the stomach
   8. For snakebite
   9. Again, for snakebite
   10. For intestinal worms
   11. For a hard place on the body
   12. For quartan fever
   13. For gout and sore tendons
   14. For tertian fever
   15. For two-day fever
   16. For infected wounds
   17. For swollen feet on a trip
   18. For a sore on the nose or cheek
   19. For strange pustules on the nose
   20. For mouth injuries
   21. For bite of a mad dog
   22. For daily internal weakness

3. The *pentafilon* plant, which is **cinquefoil**
   1. For joints that ache or are diseased
   2. For stomach pain
   3. For aching mouth, tongue, and throat
   4. For headache
   5. For severe nosebleed
   6. For aching midriff
   7. For snakebite
   8. For burns
   9. If you want to stop ulcerous sores from spreading

4. The *uermenaca* plant, which is **vervain**
    1. For wounds, carbuncles, and swollen glands[1]
    2. Again, for swollen glands
    3. For those who have clogged veins so that blood cannot get to the genitals and for those who cannot keep their food down
    4. For liver pain
    5. For bladder stones
    6. For headache
    7. For snakebite
    8. For poisonous spider bite
    9. For bite of a mad dog
    10. For fresh wounds
    11. For snakebite
5. The *sinphoniaca* plant, which is **henbane**
    1. For earache
    2. For swollen knees or calves or other swellings on the body
    3. For toothache
    4. For genital soreness or swelling
    5. For painful breasts
    6. For sore feet
    7. For lung disease
6. The *uiperina* plant, which is **bistort** or **snakeweed**
    1. For snakebite
7. The *ueneria* plant, which is **sweet flag**
    1. To prevent bees' swarming
    2. For inability to urinate
8. The plant *pes leonis*, which is **lion's foot** or **lady's mantle**
    1. For being under an evil spell
9. The *scelerata* plant, which is **celery-leaved crowfoot**
    1. For wounds and carbuncles
    2. For swellings and warts
10. The *batracion* plant, which is **buttercup** or **meadow crowfoot**
    1. For lunacy
    2. For darkened sores
11. The *artemesia* plant, which is **mugwort**
    1. For a sore abdomen
    2. For sore feet
12. The *artemesia tagantes* plant, which is the second kind of mugwort, called **tansy**

---

1. Beginning here, the numbering in C and DeV differ very slightly on some items; DeV's numbering is retained. This should not pose a problem when comparing C with the current version, because they are at most one number different from each other.

1. For bladder pain
2. For sore thighs
3. For sore and swollen tendons
4. For severe gout
5. For fever

13. The *artemesia leptefilos* plant, which is a third kind of mugwort, called **roman wormwood**
    1. For stomachache
    2. For trembling tendons

14. The *lapatium* plant, which is **dock**
    1. For swellings that grow on the genitals

15. The *dracontea* plant, which is **dragonwort**
    1. For snakebite
    2. For broken bones

16. The *satyrion* plant, which is **orchis** or **wild orchid**
    1. For painful wounds
    2. For eye pain

17. The *gentiana* plant, which is **yellow gentian**
    1. For snakebite

18. The *orbicularis* plant, which is **cyclamen** or **sowbread**
    1. For hair loss
    2. For irritable bowels
    3. For pain in the spleen

19. The *proserpinaca* plant, which is **knotgrass**
    1. For spitting blood
    2. For pain in the sides
    3. For sore nipples
    4. For eye pain
    5. For earache
    6. For diarrhea

20. The *aristolochia* plant, which is **heartwort** or **birthwort**
    1. Against strong poison
    2. For bad fevers
    3. For sore nostrils
    4. For a chilled person
    5. For snakebite
    6. For an upset child
    7. For a sore growing on the nose

21. The *nasturcium* plant, which is **watercress** or **garden cress**
    1. For hair falling out
    2. For head sores accompanied by dandruff and itching
    3. For soreness in the body
    4. For swellings
    5. For warts

22. The *hieribulbum* plant, which is **meadow saffron** or **tassel hyacinth**
    1. For sore joints
    2. If pimples grow on a woman's nose
23. The *apollinaris* plant[2]
    1. For sore hands
24. The *camemelon* plant, which is **camomile**
    1. For eye pain
25. The *chamedris* plant, which is **wall germander**
    1. If anything is bruised
    2. For snakebite
    3. For gout
26. The *chameælee* plant, which is **wild teasel**
    1. For liver sickness
    2. For poison
    3. For dropsy
27. The *chamepithys* plant, which is **ground-pine**
    1. For wounds
    2. For abdominal pain
28. The *chamedafne* plant, which is **spurge** or **figwort**
    1. To move the intestines
29. The *ostriago* plant[3] or **madder**
    1. For everything producing sores on people
30. The *brittanica* plant, which is **red dock** or **great water dock**
    1. For mouth sores
    2. Again, for mouth sores
    3. For toothache
    4. To move clogged intestines
    5. For pain in the side
31. The *lactuca* plant, which is **wild lettuce**
    1. For sore eyes
    2. Again, for dim eyes
32. The *agrimonia* plant, which is **agrimony**
    1. For sore eyes
    2. For sore abdomen
    3. For ulcerous sores and wounds
    4. For snakebite
    5. For warts
    6. For soreness of the spleen
    7. If you want to cut something from the body
    8. For a blow from iron

---

2. D'A = no English name. Bierbaumer, DeV, C = Lily of the Valley. Old English = *glofwyrt*.
3. Bierbaumer, DeV = wayfaring tree. C = lithewort.

33. The *astularegia* plant, which is **asphodel**
    1. For leg-shank pain
    2. For liver pain
34. The *lapatium* plant, which is **dock**
    1. If body stiffness occurs
35. The *centauria maior* plant[4]
    1. For liver disease
    2. For wounds and ulcerous sores
36. The *centauria minor* plant, which is **common** or **lesser centaury**
    1. For snakebite
    2. For eye pain
    3. Again, for eye pain
    4. For nerve spasms
    5. For tasting poison
    6. For anal worms
37. The *personacia* plant, which is **burdock**[5]
    1. For wounds and snakebite
    2. For fevers
    3. For ulcerous sores on wounds
    4. For pain in the abdomen
    5. For bite of a mad dog
    6. For fresh wounds
38. The *fraga* plant, which is **wild strawberry**
    1. For pain of the spleen
    2a. For shortness of breath (asthma)
    2b. For abdominal pain
39. The *hibiscus* plant, which is **marshmallow**
    1. For gout
    2. For any accumulation of diseased matter growing on the body
40. The *ippirus* plant, which is **horsetail**
    1. For dysentery
    2. For coughing up blood
41. The *malfa erratica* plant, which is **mallow**
    1. For bladder pain
    2. For sore tendons
    3. For pain in the side
    4. For fresh wounds

---

4. D'A says no English name. C, DeV, Bierbaumer = *Blackstonia perfoliata*, yellow wort.
5. D'A explains that the Old English word denotes *Beta vulagaris,* or beet.
6. D'A notes controversy over the identification of this plant. C, DeV, Bierbaumer = *Cynoglossum officinale*, hound's-tongue.

42. The *buglossa* plant, which is **alkanet**[6]
    1. For tertian or quartan fever
    2. For shortness of breath (asthma)
43. The *bulbiscillitica* plant, which is **sea onion** or **squill**
    1. For dropsy
    2. For painful joints
    3. For the disease the Greeks call *paranichias* (chilblains)
    4. If one cannot quench the thirst of a person with dropsy
44. The *cotiledon* plant, which is **navelwort**
    1. For swellings
45. The *gallicrus* plant, which is **cockspur grass**
    1. For dog bite
46. The *prassion* plant, which is **horehound**
    1. For a head cold and for violent coughing
    2. For stomachache
    3. For worms around the anus
    4. For sore joints and for swellings
    5. For tasting poison
    6. For scabs and impetigo
    7. For lung disease
    8. For every body stiffness
47. The *xifion* plant, which is **gladiolus**
    1. For strange carbuncles growing on the body
    2. For a fractured skull and poisoned bones
48. The *gallitricus* plant, which is **true maidenhair**
    1. If swellings harm a virgin
    2. For hair loss
49. The *temolus* plant, which is **garlic**
    1. For pain in the womb
50. The *æliotrophus* plant, which is **heliotrope**[7]
    1. For all poisons
    2. For flux
51. The *gryas* plant, which is **madder**
    1. For aching legs and broken bones
    2. For every pain that hurts the body
52. The *politricus* plant or **common maidenhair**[8]
    1. For abdominal pain and to promote hair growth
53. The *malochinagria* plant, which is **asphodel**[9]
    1. For swollen abdomen
    2. For abdominal flux

7. Bierbaumer, DeV = cat's-ear.
8. Bierbaumer, C = *Campanula trachelium*, yellow clover.
9. DeV, Bierbaumer = sweet woodruff.

54. The *metoria* plant, which is **white poppy**
    2. For pain in the temples[10]
    3. For sleeplessness
55. The *oenantes* plant[11]
    1. For inability to urinate
    2. If anyone coughs very strongly
56. The *narcisus* plant, which is **narcissus** or **throatwort**
    1. For sores that are growing on people
57. The *splenion* plant, which is **spleenwort** or **figwort**
    1. For pain in the spleen
58. The *polion* plant[12]
    1. For insanity
59. The *uictoriola* plant, which is **butcher's-broom**
    1. For gout and stomachache
60. The *confirma* plant, which is **comfrey**
    1. For menstruation
    2. If anything internal is ruptured
    3. For stomachache
61. The *asterion* plant[13]
    1. For epilepsy
62. The *leporis pes* plant, which is **hare's-foot clover**
    1. For constipation
63. The *dictamnus* plant[14]
    1. If a woman has a stillborn child inside her
    2. For wounds
    3. For snakebite
    4. For tasting poison
    5. Again, for fresh wounds
64. The *solago maior* plant, which is *heliotropion*[15]
    1. Again, for snakebite
65. The *solago minor* plant, which is *aeliotropion*[16]
    1. For worms around the anus
66. The *peonia* plant[17]
    1. For lunacy
    2. For sciatica

---

10. The contents entry corresponding to remedy 1 in the text of the *Herbarium* is missing; hence the numbering here starts at 2.
11. Dropwort.
12. Sage-leaved germander or wood sage.
13. Aster. C, DeV = chickweed.
14. Dittany of Crete or white dittany.
15. Heliotrope.
16. D'A = no English name. C, DeV = croton.
17. Peony.

67.   The *peristereon* plant, which is **vervain** or **gipsy-wort**
    1.   For dog's bark
    2.   For all poisons
68.   The *bryonia* plant, which is **bryony**
    1.   For pain in the spleen
69.   The *nymfete* plant[18]
    1.   For diarrhea, again for diarrhea
    2.   Again, for abdominal pain
    3.   For diarrhea
70.   The *crision* plant, which is **thistle**
    1.   For sore throat
71.   The *isatis* plant[19]
    2.   For snakebite
72.   The *scordea* plant[20]
    1.   Again, for snakebite
    2.   For sore joints
    3.   For fever
73.   The *uerbascus* plant, which is **great mullein**
How Mercury gave the plant to Iulixe
    1.   Against all bad encounters
    2.   For gout
74.   The *heraclea* plant[21]
    1.   If one wants to travel a long way and does not want to fear robbers
75.   The *cælidonia* plant, which is **greater celandine**
    1.   For dimness and soreness of the eyes
    2.   Again, for dimming eyesight
    3.   For swellings
    4.   For headache
    5.   If one is burned
76.   The *solata* plant, which is **black nightshade**[22]
    1.   For swellings
    2.   For earache
    3.   For toothache
    4.   For a bloody nose
77.   The *senecio* plant, which is **common groundsel**
    1.   For wounds, even if they are old
    2.   For a blow from something iron
    3.   For gout

---

18. White water lily.
19. Woad.
20. Water germander.
21. D'A = no English name. C, DeV = star thistle.
22. C, DeV, Bierbaumer = deadly nightshade.

      4.   For sore loins

78.   The *felix* plant, which is **fern**
1. For wounds
2. For rupture in a young man

79.   The *gramen* plant, which is **couch grass**[23]
1. For pain in the spleen

80.   The *gladiolum* plant, which is **iris**
1. For bladder pain and inability to urinate
2. For pain of the spleen
3. For abdominal pain and breast pain

81.   The *rosmarinum* plant, which is **rosemary**
1. For toothache

  2., 3. For ill people and for itching
4. For liver and abdominal disease
5. For fresh wounds

82.   The *pastinaca siluatica* plant, which is **wild carrot** or **parsnip**
1. For difficult childbirth
2. For a woman's cleansing

83.   The *perdicalis* plant, which is **pellitory-of-the-wall**
1. For gout and ulcerous sores

84.   The *mercurialis* plant, which is **mercury**
1. For abdominal hardening
2. If a great deal of water gets in the ears

85.   The *radiola* plant, which is **polypody**
1. For headache

86.   The *sparagiagrestis* plant, which is **asparagus**
1. For pain or swelling of the bladder
2. For toothache
3. For sore veins
4. For a case where one person puts another under a spell by ill will

87.   The *sabine* plant, which is **savine**
1. For painful joints and foot swelling
2. For headache
3. For carbuncles

88.   The *canis caput*, which is the **small snapdragon**
1. For soreness and swelling of the eyes

89.   The *erusti* plant, which is **blackberry** or **bramble**
1. For earache
2. For menstruation
3. For heart pain
4. For fresh wounds

---

23. C, DeV, Bierbaumer = quitch.

     5.   For pain in the joints

     6.   For snakebite

90.   The *millefolium* plant, which is **yarrow**

     1.   For a blow from something iron and tells that Achilles discovered the plant

     2.   For toothache

     3.   For wounds

     4.   For swellings

     5.   For difficulty in urinating

     6.   If a wound has grown cold on a person

     7.   If the head breaks out in rashes or for strange swellings on the face

     8.   For the same

     9.   If the veins are hardened or a person has difficulty digesting food

     10.   For intestinal and abdominal pain

     11.   If hiccoughs trouble one

     12.   For headache

     13.   For bite of the snake called *spalangius*

     14.   Again, for snakebite

     15.   For bite of a mad dog

     16.   For snakebite

91.   The *ruta* plant, which is **rue**

     1.   For nosebleed

     2.   For swellings

     3.   For stomachache

     4.   For pain and swelling of the eyes

     5.   For forgetfulness

     6.   For dimness of the eyes

     7.   For headache

92.   The *mentastrus* plant, which is **horsemint**

     1.   For earache

     2.   For itchy skin conditions

93.   The *ebulus* plant, which is **dwarf elder** or **danewort**

     1.   For stones in the bladder

     2.   For snakebite

     3.   For dropsy

94.   The *pollegium* plant, which is **pennyroyal**

     1.   For abdominal pain

     2.   For stomach pain

     3.   For genital itching

     4.   Again, for abdominal pain

     5.   For tertian fever

     6.   If a stillborn child is in a woman's abdomen

      7. For seasickness
      8. For bladder pain and the stones growing there
      9. If anyone suffers from pain around the heart or chest
    10. For a cramp
    11. For stomach and abdominal swelling
    12. For pain of the spleen
    13. For pain of the loins or thighs

95. The *nepitamon* plant, which is **nepata**[24]
      1. For snakebite

96. The *peucedana* plant, which is **sulphurweed** or **hog's fennel**
      1. Again, for snakebite
      2. For witlessness of the mind

97. The *hinnula campana* plant, which is **elecampane**
      1. For bladder pain
      2. For toothache and loose teeth
      3. For worms around the anus

98. The *cynoglossa* plant, which is **hound's-tongue**[25]
      1. For snakebite
      2. For quartan fever
      3. For poor hearing

99. The *saxifragia* plant, which is **saxifrage**
      1. For stones in the bladder

100. The *hedera nigra* plant, which is **ivy**
      1. Again, for stones in the bladder
      2. For headache
      3. For pain in the spleen
      4. For bite of the spider called *spalangiones*
      5. Again, to heal wounds
      6. For evil-smelling nostrils
      7. For poor hearing
      8. To prevent a headache from the sun

101. The *serpillus* plant, which is **wild thyme**
      1. For headache
      2. Again, for headache
      3. For burns

102. The *absinthius* plant, which is **wormwood**
      1. For bruises and other sores
      2. For ringworm

---

24. C, DeV, Bierbaumer = catmint.
25. D'A notes here that the Old English word denotes narrow-leaved plantain.
26. Sage.

103. The *salfia* plant[26]
    1. For genital itching
    2. Again, for anal itching
104. The *coliandra* plant, which is **coriander**
    1. For worms
    2. So a woman can give birth quickly
105. The *porclaca* plant[27]
    1. For excessive flow of semen
106. The *cerefolia* plant, which is **chervil**
    1. For stomachache
107. The *sisimbrius* plant[28]
    1. For bladder pain and inability to urinate
108. The *olisatra* plant[29]
    1. Again, for bladder pain and painful urination
109. The *lilium* plant, which is **lily**
    1. For snakebite
    2. For swellings
110. The *tytymallus* plant, which is **caper-spurge**
    1. For abdominal pain
    2. For warts
    3. For skin irritations
111. The *carduus siluaticus* plant, which is **sow-thistle**
    1. For stomachache
    2. So that you will not fear encountering any evil
112. The *lupinus montanus* plant[30]
    1. For worms about the anus
    2. For the same in children
113. The *lactyrida* plant, which is **spurge laurel**
    1. For constipation
114. The *lactuca leporina* plant, which is **great chondrilla** or **lettuce**
    1. For feverishness
115. The *cucumeris siluatica* plant, which is **cucumber**[31]
    1. For sore joints and gout
    2. If a child is born prematurely or misshapen
116. The *cannaue silfatica* plant[32]
    1. For a sore chest
    2. For chill burns

---

27. Purslane.
28. Brook or water mint.
29. Alexanders or horse parsley.
30. Lupin.
31. D'A specifies "squirting cucumber," a plant that grows near water in warm places.
32. Hemp.

117. The *ruta montana* plant, which is **wild rue**
    1. For dim eyesight
    2. For a sore chest
    3. For liver pain
    4. For inability to urinate
    5. For snakebite
118. The *eptafilon* plant, which is **tormentil**
    1. For gout
119. The *ocimus* plant, which is **basil**
    1. For headache
    2. For eye pain and swelling
    3. For kidney pain
120. The *apium* plant, which is **wild celery**
    1. For eye pain and swelling
121. The *hedera crysocantes* plant, which is **ivy**
    1. For dropsy
122. The *menta* plant, which is **mint**
    1. For impetigo and pimples
    2. For bad scars and wounds
123. The *anetum* plant, which is **dill**
    1. For genital itching and pain
    2. If a woman suffers from the same
    3. For headache
124. The *origanum* plant, which is **wild** or **sweet marjoram**
    1. For gout, liver disease, and shortness of breath
    2. For coughs
125. The *semperuiuus* plant, which is **houseleek**
    1. For all painful accumulations of fluids
126. The *fenuculus* plant, which is **fennel**
    1. For coughs and shortness of breath
    2. For bladder pain
127. The *erifion* plant, which is **rue**
    1. For lung disease
128. The *sinfitus albus* plant[33]
    1. For menstruation
129. The *petroselinum* plant, which is **parsley**
    1. For snakebite
    2. For nerve pain
130. The *brassica siluatica* plant, which is **cabbage** or **colewort**
    1. For all swellings
    2. For pain in the side
    3. For gout

---

33. Comfrey.

131. The *basilisca* plant, which is **sweet basil**
    1. For all types of snakes
132. The *mandragora* plant[34]
    1. For headache
    2. For earache
    3. For gout
    4. For insanity
    5. Again, for nerve spasms
    6. If anyone sees great evil in the house
133. The *lychanis stephanice* plant, which is **campion**
    1. For all types of snakes
134. The *action* plant[35]
    1. If one coughs up blood and phlegm
    2. For pain in the joints
135. The *abrotanus* plant, which is **southernwood**
    1. For shortness of breath, sciatica, and pain when urinating
    2. For pain in the side
    3. For poison and snakebite
    4. Again, for snakebite
    5. For eye pain
136. The *sion* plant, which is **water parsnip**
    1. For stones in the bladder
    2. For dysentery and for diarrhea
137. The *eliotropus* plant, which is **white heliotrope**
    1. For all snakebites
    2. For worms that bother the area around the anus
    3. For warts
138. The *spreritis* plant[36]
    1. For fever chills
    2. For the bite of a mad dog
    3. For pain of the spleen
139. The *aizos minor* plant[37]
    1. For impetigo and eye pain and gout
    2. For headache
    3. For bite of the snake named *spalangiones*
    4. For dysentery and diarrhea and if worms trouble the intestines
    5. Again, for any disease of the eye
140. The *elleborus* plant, which is **white hellebore**
    1. About the power of this plant

---

34. Mandrake.
35. Burdock.
36. Field marigold.
37. Stonecrop.

       2.   For diarrhea

       3.   For diseases and for all evil

141.   The *buoptalmon* plant[38]

       1.   For any bad boils

       2.   For damage to the body

142.   The *tribulus* plant, which is **land caltrop**

       1.   For a very hot body

       2.   For swelling and foulness of the mouth and throat

       3.   For bladder stones

       4.   For snakebite

       5.   For drinking poison

       6.   For fleas

143.   The *coniza* plant[39]

       1.   For snakebite, to put gnats, mosquitoes, and fleas to flight, and for wounds

      2., 3.   To purify a woman's womb and if a woman cannot give birth

       4.   For fever chills

       5.   For headache

144.   The *tricnos manicos* plant, which is **thorn-apple** or **datura**

       1.   For impetigo (teter)

       2.   For impetigo

       3.   For headache and stomach burn and pimples

       4.   For earache

145.   The *glycyrida* plant[40]

       1.   For a dry fever

       2.   For chest, liver, and bladder pain

       3.   For diseases of the mouth

146.   The *strutius* plant[41]

       1.   For inability to urinate

       2.   For liver disease and shortness of breath and bad coughs and diarrhea

       3.   For bladder stones

       4.   For skin irritations

       5.   For bad swellings

147.   The *aizon* plant[42]

       1.   For a sore-ruptured body, putrefaction, eye pain and heat, and burns

       3.   For snakebites (2 is missing)

       4.   For dysentery and intestinal worms

---

38. Oxeye daisy or marguerite.
39. Fleabane or spikenard.
40. Licorice.
41. Soapwort.
42. Orpine.

148. The *samsuchon* plant, which is **sweet marjoram**
    1. For dropsy and inability to urinate and diarrhea
    2. For carbuncles and skin eruptions
    3. For scorpion sting
    4. For heat and swelling of the eyes
149. The *stecas* plant[43]
    1. For chest pain
150. The *thyaspis* plant[44]
    1. For all painful swellings of the intestines and for menstruation
151. The *polis* plant, which is **wood sage** or **sage-leaved germander**
    1. For snakebite
    2. For dropsy
    3. For pain of the spleen, to chase away snakes, and for fresh wounds
152. The *ypericon* plant, which is **St. John's wort**
    1. To stimulate urination and menstruation
    2. For quartan fever
    3. For swelling and aching of the leg shanks
153. The *acantaleuca* plant[45]
    1. For coughing up blood and stomach pain
    2. To stimulate urination
    3. For toothache and bad bruises
    4. For cramps and snakebite
154. The *acanton* plant, which is **Scotch thistle**
    1. To move the intestines and urine
    2. For lung disease and for any evil
155. The *guiminon* plant, which is **caraway** or **cumin**
    1. For stomachache
    2. For shortness of breath and snakebite
    3. For tenderness and heat of the abdomen
    4. For nosebleed
156. The *camelleon alba* plant, which is **carline thistle**
    1. If intestinal worms trouble one about the anus
    2. For dropsy and difficulty in urinating
157. The *scolymbos* plant[46]
    1. For foul-smelling armpits and for a foul smell anywhere on the body
158. The *iris Yllyrica* plant[47]
    1. For deep coughs and to move the intestines

---

43. French lavender.
44. Shepherd's purse.
45. Globe thistle.
46. Artichoke.
47. German iris.

2a.   For snakebite

2b.   To stimulate a woman's menses

3.   For boils and glandular swellings and all bad swellings

4.   For headache

159.   The *elleborus albus* plant[48]

1.   For liver disease and all poisons

160.   The *delfinion* plant[49]

1.   For quartan fever

161.   The *acios* plant[50]

1.   For snakebite and sore thighs

162.   The *centimorbia* plant[51]

1.   If the back of a horse is injured at the shoulder and is open

163.   The *scordios* plant[52]

1,2.   To stimulate urine, for snakebite, for all poisons, and stomachache

3.   For phlegm in the chest

4.   For gout

5.   For fresh wounds

164.   The *ami* plant, which is **bishop's-weed**

1a.   To move the intestines, to stimulate urination, and for the bite of wild animals

1b.   For spots on the body

2.   For discoloration or lack of color on the body

165.   The *uiola* plant, which is **wallflower**

1.   For pain and inflammation of the womb

2.   For a variety of rectal disorders

3.   For canker sores in the mouth

4.   To stimulate the menses

5.   For pain of the spleen

166.   The *uiola purpurea* plant[53]

1.   For fresh wounds and also for old ones

2.   For hardening of the stomach

167.   The *zamalentition* plant[54]

1.   For all wounds

2.   For ulcerous sores

---

48. Sea onion, squill.
49. Larkspur.
50. Viper's bugloss.
51. Moneywort.
52. Barrenwort.
53. Sweet violet.
54. Unidentified.
55. Alkanet.

168. The *ancusa* plant[55]
    1. For a bad burn
169. The *psillios* plant[56]
    1. For glandular swellings and all bad swellings
    2. For a headache
170. The *cynosbatus* plant[57]
    1. For pain of the spleen
171. The *aglaofotis* plant[58]
    1. For tertian or quartan fever
    2. If stormy weather troubles one while rowing
    3. For cramps and tremors
172. The *capparis* plant, which is **caper**
    1. For pain of the spleen
173. The *eryngius* plant[59]
    1. To induce urination and menstruation and to move the intestines
    2. For a variety of abdominal diseases
    3. For swollen breasts
    4a. For scorpion sting, snakebites, and bites from a mad dog
    4b. For impetigo and gout
174. The *philantropos* plant[60]
    1. For snakebites and bite of the serpent called *spalangiones*
    2. For earache
175. The *achillea* plant[61]
    1. For fresh wounds
    2. If a woman suffers from watery discharge from the sexual organs
    3. For diarrhea
176. The *rincus* plant[62]
    1. To turn away hail and storms
177. The *polloten* plant, which is **black horehound**
    1. For dog bite
    2. For wounds
178. The *urtica* plant, which is **nettle**
    1. For chilled wounds
    2. For swellings
    3. If any part of the body is struck
    4. For pain in the thighs
    5. For putrefied wounds

---

56. Fleawort.
57. Sweet briar or eglantine.
58. Peony.
59. Sea holly or eryngo.
60. Cleavers or goosegrass.
61. Yarrow.
62. Castor-oil plant.

      6.   For menstruation

      7.   So that cold will not bother you

179.   The *priapisci* plant, which is **greater periwinkle**

      For possession by demons, for snakes, wild animals, poisons, for any threats, envy, terror, so you will have grace, so you will be happy and comfortable

180.   The *litosperimon* plant[63]

      1.   For bladder stones

181.   The *stavisacre* plant[64]

      1.   For bad fluids in the body

      2.   For scaly skin and scabs

      3.   For toothache and sore gums

182.   The *gorgonion* plant[65]

      1.   For bad swelling of the feet

183.   The *milotis* plant[66]

      1.   For dimness of the eyes

      2.   For muscle spasms

184.   The *bulbus* plant[67]

      1.   For swellings and gout and any injury

      2a.   For dropsy

      2b.   For dog bite, if one sweats, for stomachache

      3.   For wounds, scaly skin, and pimples

      4.   For tenderness and ruptures of the abdomen

185.   The *colocynthisagria* plant, which is **bitter cucumber**

      1.   To move the bowels

Remedies

1. Wood Betony (*Stachys officinalis*), *betonica, Biscopwyrt*[68]

    1.   This plant, which is named *betonica* [betony], is grown in meadows, on cleared hilly land,[69] and in sheltered[70] places; it is good both for one's soul and one's body; it protects a person from dreadful night-

---

63. Common gromwell.

64. Stavisacre or lousewort.

65. D'A = unidentified. C, DeV, Bierbaumer = field eryngo.

66. Melilot.

67. Tassel hyacinth.

68. Each heading provides: (1) the modern English plant name, (2) official botanical name, (3) medieval Latin or Greek name, and (4) the Old English name. In the remedies, wherever the plant name in the original was Latin or Greek, it is retained here and set in italics; the modern English name follows in square brackets. Where an Old English plant name was used in the manuscript, it is translated directly into modern English. The entire chapter on betony was originally a separate work titled *De herba vettonica liber,* as mentioned earlier.

69. *on clænum dunlandum.* C = clean downlands. DOE = *dun* = hill. *clænsian* = to cleanse, purify.

70. *gefriþedum* = sheltered. C = shady.

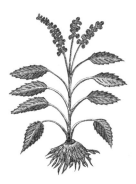

mares[71] and from terrifying visions and dreams. This plant is very wholesome and so you must gather it in the month of August without using a tool made of iron; and when you have gathered it, shake off the dirt[72] so that none sticks to it and then dry it very thoroughly in the shade. Then, together with all its roots, make it into a powder;[73] then use it and taste it when you need to.

2. If a person's skull is shattered, take the same plant, *betonica* [betony]; shred[74] it and pound it into a powder. Then take two coins' weight of it and drink it in hot beer. The skull will heal very quickly after the drink.[75]

3. For eye pain, take roots of the same plant and simmer them down in water until the liquid is reduced by two-thirds.[76] Bathe the eyes with the water, take the leaves of the same plant, crush them, and lay them on the face over the eyes.

4. For earache, take the leaves of this same plant when it is greenest, gently boil them in water, and press the juice out,[77] and after it has stood for a time, warm it up again and use a piece of wool to drip it into the ear.

5. For dimness of the eyes, take one coin's weight of this same plant, *betonica* [betony], and boil gently in water. Give it to a person to drink on an empty stomach, because it dilutes the part of the blood from which the dimness arises.

71. *nihtgengum* = evil night spirit. C = monstrous nocturnal visitors. Nightmare captures this meaning, particularly in view of the uses following for betony.
72. *molde, -an* = dust, earth, etc. C = mold
73. *gewyrc to duste*. C = reduce it to dust. In this context dust is misleading.
74. *scearfian* = scrape, shred. C = scrape, but shred would make more sense here before the plant (possibly dried) was made into a powder.
75. This is a radical departure from the Latin text, and from Dioscorides, in which the pounded betony is put on the broken skull to heal the fractured bones. Might this Anglo-Saxon cure instead be for migrane headache, when the head indeed feels *tobroken*?
76. *seoð on wætere to þriddan dæle*. C = boil it down to the third part. Modern usage is to reduce liquid by so much, usually by simmering (not boiling) a long time.
77. *wring þæt wos* (*wos* is juice). C = wring the wash.

6. For watery eyes, take the same plant, *betonica* [betony], and give it to the patient to eat. It helps and will make the eyes' sharpness clear.

7. For excessive flow of blood from the nose, take the same plant, *betonica* [betony], pound it, and mix with it a bit of salt. Then take as much as you can with two fingers, work it into a ball, and put it into the nostrils.

8. For toothache, take the same plant, *betonica* [betony], and simmer it down rapidly by two-thirds in aged wine. It greatly heals the toothache and swelling.

9. For pain in the side,[78] take three coins' weight of the same plant; simmer in aged wine. Grind twenty-seven peppercorns and add them to it. Drink three cupfuls at night, on an empty stomach.

10. For pain in the loins, take the three coins' weight of the same, *betonica* [betony], and seventeen peppercorns; grind them together and boil gently in aged wine. Give three cupfuls to drink warm, at night, on an empty stomach.

11. For stomach pain, take two[79] coins' weight of the same plant, boil gently in water, then give it warm to the person to drink. The stomach pain will diminish and be soothed, so that soon there will not be any pain.

12. If a person is constipated,[80] take this same plant in warm water at night on an empty stomach. The person will be well in the space of three nights.

13. In case blood gushes up through a person's mouth, take three coins' weight of the same plant and three cupfuls of cold goat's milk. The person will be very quickly healed.

14. If a person does not want to be drunk, then take the *betonica* [betony] plant before drinking.

15. If a boil appears on the face, take one coin's weight, pound with aged fat, lay on the place where the boil wants to settle, and it will soon be healed.

16. If a person is ruptured inside or the body is sore, take four coins' weight of the *betonica* [betony] plant, boil it gently in wine. Drink it at night on an empty stomach; then the body will soon be relieved.

17. If a person becomes tired from much riding or much walking, take one coin's weight of the *betonica* [betony] plant and simmer it in sweet wine. Drink three full cups at night on an empty stomach. The person will quickly not be weary.

---

78. *Wiþ sidan sare.* C = for sore of side.
79. *twega* = two. C = three to agree with the Latin original!
80. *Gif mannes innoð to fæst sy. innoð* = intestines, abdomen, sometimes womb. *Fæstnyss* is constipation. C = if a mans inwards be too fast.

18.   If a person is not well inside or is nauseated, then you take two coins' weight of the *betonica* [betony] plant and one ounce of honey. Thoroughly and gently boil this in beer, drink three cupfuls at night on an empty stomach, and the insides will quickly open up.

19.   If you want your food to digest easily, take three coins' weight of the *betonica* [betony] plant and one ounce of honey. Simmer the plant until it thickens, then drink it in two cupfuls of water.

20.   If a person cannot keep food down and vomits when he swallows, take four coins' weight of the *betonica* [betony] plant and boiled honey, then make four little pills from it. Eat one, take one in hot water, and then two in wine. Then swallow three cupfuls of water.

21.   For abdominal pain, or if one is swollen, take the *betonica* [betony] plant, crumble it very fine in wine, lay some around the stomach, and eat some of it. That will quickly bring recovery.

22.   If anyone drinks poison, let him take three coins' weight of that same plant and four cups of wine; gently boil them together, then drink them, and then the person will vomit up the poison.

23.   If a snake bites someone, let him take four coins' weight of the same plant crumbled very small and gently boil in wine. Then lay it on the wound and also drink a great deal of it; then you will be able to heal the bite of any snake.

24.   Again, for snakebite, take one coin's weight of that same plant, crumble it into red wine (ensure there are three cups of wine), and smear the wound with the plants and the wine; it will soon be healthy.

25.   For bite of a mad dog, take the *betonica* [betony] plant, pound it very small, and lay it on the wound.

26.   If your throat or any part of your neck is sore, take the same plant, pound it very small, make it into a poultice, and lay it on the neck; it will clean it up both inside and out.

27.   For sore loins, and if a person's thighs ache, take two coins' weight of the same plant, boil it gently in beer, and give to the person to drink.

28.   If a person is feverish and suffering from being very hot, give the plant in warm water, definitely not in beer. The soreness in the loins and the thighs will get better very quickly.[81]

29.   For gout, take the same plant, simmer it down in water by two-thirds, pound the plant, lay it on the feet, and rub it on. Drink the juice. You will find recovery and excellent health.

---

81. Such a remedy, containing a reference to a condition mentioned just before it, without being explicit, is not unusual in this work. The presence of a fever generally calls for a slightly different approach.

2. Common Plantain (*Plantago maior L.*), *arniglosa, Wægbræde*

1. If the head aches or is sore, take the roots of the common plantain plant and bandage them to the neck; the soreness will leave the head.
2. If the stomach is sore, take the juice of the greater plantain plant, ensure that it is clear,[82] and drink it. Then with a great deal of nausea, the soreness will depart. If it happens that the abdomen is swollen, shred the plant, lay it on the abdomen, and the swelling will disappear[83] quickly.
3. For pain in the abdomen, take plantain juice, put it in some kind of ale,[84] and drink a great deal of it; it heals internally and purges the stomach and the small intestines wondrously well.
4. Again, if someone has a swollen abdomen,[85] simmer the plantain at just below the boil and then eat a great deal of it; the abdomen will go down quickly.
5. Again, if blood runs out a person's anus, take plantain juice and give it to the person to drink; it will quickly stop.
6. If a person is wounded, take plantain seed, grind it into a powder, and sprinkle it on the wound; it will quickly be well. If the body is afflicted anywhere with hot inflammations, pound the same plant and lay it on there; then the body will cool down and heal.

---

82. *genime wegbræden seaw ðære wyrte, gedo þæt hio blacu sy.* C= take the juice of waybread the wort, and contrive that it be lukewarm. Cockayne says in a note that the word *blacu* (pale) is a scribal error for *wlacu* (lukewarm), because *hio* refers to *wyrte* (f.), not to *seaw*, a neuter noun. However, the error could be in the adjective ending; after all, *wyrte* is the closest word to *blacu*. Moreover, Culpepper advises clarifying the juice of the greater plantain plant before giving it to drink. No matter the literal construction, and allowing for vague referents in Old English, I would argue that clear (clarified) juice is intended here.

83. *fordwineð.* C = dwindle.

84. *do on sumes cynnes ealo* (C says it is *cald*, not *ealo* in MS V). C = put it on cold of some kind.

85. C = a man be overgrown in wamb.

7. If you want to soften a person's stomach, take the plant and simmer it in vinegar. Pour the liquid and the cooked plant into some wine, then drink this at night on an empty stomach, always one cup as a full dose.[86]

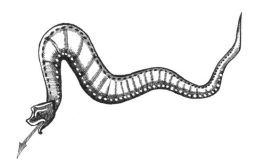

8. For snakebite, take the plantain plant, crush it into some wine, and eat it.

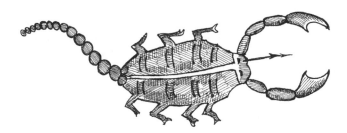

9. For the bite of a scorpion, take plantain roots and bandage them onto the person; it is believed that this will be of good service.
10. If intestinal worms trouble a person, take plantain juice (pound and wring the plant [to get the juice]), and give it to the person to drink. Take the same plant, pound it well, lay it on the anus and fasten it there tightly.

---

86. C = always one cup for a discharge.

11. If anyone's body develops a hard lump,[87] take the plantain plant, mix in unsalted grease, make it into a poultice,[88] and put it onto the hard spot; it will quickly soften and heal.

12. If quartan fever afflicts a person, take the juice of that plant, mix it with water, and give it to the person to drink two hours before he expects the fever;[89] then there is hope that it will benefit greatly.

13. For gout and for sore tendons, take the leaves of plantain, mix them with salt, and put this on the feet and the tendons; that is a certain remedy.

14. For tertain fever, take three plantain roots[90] and mix them in water or wine; give this to the person before the fever comes to drink at night on an empty stomach.

15. For fever that returns every twenty-four hours, pound the same plant very fine and give it to the person to drink in ale; it is believed that this helps.

16. For infected wounds,[91] take the plantain plant and mix it into unsalted grease. Put this onto the wound, and it will heal quickly.

17. If a person's feet swell during a journey, take the plantain plant and mix it in vinegar. Bathe and smear the feet with it; they will quickly become less swollen.

18. If a sore develops on someone's nose or cheek, take plantain juice, wring it into soft wool, and lay it on the sore. Let it lie there nine nights; it will heal up soon after that.

19. For any strange pustules that arise on the nose, take plantain seed, dry it, grind it and mix it with grease, put a little salt into it, and soak it with wine.[92] Smear it on the nose; it will become smooth and heal.

20. For an injury to the mouth, take plantain leaves and their juice, mix them together, have them in your mouth for a long time, and then eat the root.

21. If a mad dog bites a person, take the same herb, pound it fine, and apply it; it will quickly heal.

---

87. *licoma sy ahearded.* C = a mans body be hardened. It is unlikely the whole body would be hard; instead, this remedy would soften a hard lump somewhere on the body. This is a use Culpepper lists for plantain.

88. *to clame.* C = work it to clam (a clammy substance). Several remedies call for "grease without salt," which is translated here as unsalted grease. Bacon grease and other greases made from fat that was cured in salt would have been salty, whereas butter and unsalted fats would have been free of it (but would perish sooner).

89. Quartan fever recurrs every seventy-two hours. The Anglo-Saxon has *feorðan dages fefer.*

90. *feofre þe ðe þriddan dæge on becymeð,* or tertain fever, which occurs every thirty-six hours. Cockayne translates the part of the plant to use as plantain *sprouts,* but root is also the meaning of *cyðas* and it makes more sense in this context.

91. *wunda hatunge.* C = heats of wounds.

92. DeV remarks about a curious form for the verb that is found in MS V.

22.   For a person's everyday internal weakness,[93] take plantain, mix it in wine, drink the liquid, and eat the plantain, because it is good for any kind of internal infirmity.

3. Cinquefoil (*Potentilla reptans L.*), *pentafolium, Fifleafe*

1.   If a person's joints ache or are attacked with disease, take the cinquefoil plant, pound it very small with grease and apply it without salt; it will quickly heal.

2.   For a sore stomach, take juice of the cinquefoil plant, press out two spoonfuls, and give to the person to drink; it will clear away all of the soreness.

3.   For aching in the mouth, tongue, and throat, take cinquefoil roots, boil gently in water, and give to the person to drink; it will clear the inside of the mouth, and the ache will lessen.

4.   For headache, take the cinquefoil plant, mark around it three times with the little finger and with the thumb,[94] then pull it up from the ground, grind it into small pieces, and bandage it onto the head. The ache will lessen.

5.   If blood runs very fast out of a person's nose, give him cinquefoil to drink in wine and smear the head with it; then the bleeding will quickly stop.

6.   If a person's stomach aches, take the juice of cinquefoil, mix it with wine, and then drink three cupfuls for three mornings and evenings on an empty stomach.

7.   For snakebite, take the cinquefoil plant, mash it in wine and drink a good deal of it; it will bring recovery.[95]

8.   If a person is burned, take the cinquefoil plant, and let that person bear it on him; skillful people say[96] that it will bring recovery.

9.   If you want to stop an ulcerous sore from spreading,[97] take the cinquefoil plant, simmer it in wine and in unsalted old barrow-pig's grease. Mix it all together, make into a poultice, and lay it on the sore; then it will quickly heal. Also, you must prepare [collect and save] the plant in August.[98]

---

93. *tyddernysse* = weakness. C = every days tenderness of a man inwardly. A custom in Germany, at least until the 1960s, was to take a small shot of some kind of schnapps mid-morning to overcome "the dead time." Perhaps this was a very longstanding custom.

94. *bewrit priwa . . .* C = scratch it thrice with the least finger and the thumb. DeV = mark round (for the verb). The meaning could be to loosen the soil around the plant, since the next instruction is to pull the plant up.

95. *cymeð him to bote.* C = that will come to him for a boot (remedy).

96. *cwepað cræftige men.* C = aver crafty men.

97. *cancer ablendan.* C = blind a cancer, or prevent its discharging.

98. *Ðu scealt . . . gewyrcean þa wyrt.* C = thou shalt work up the wort.

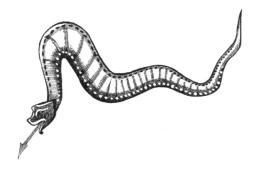

4. Vervain (*Verbena officinalis L.*), *uermenaca, Æscerote*

This plant, which is called *uermenaca* or vervain, is grown everywhere on flat and in wet lands.[99]

1. For wounds, carbuncles, and swollen glands, take the roots of the same plant and fasten them around the neck; it will benefit remarkably.
2. Again, for swollen glands, take the same plant, *uermenaca* [vervain],[100] bruise it, and lay it on the swelling; it will heal wonderfully.
3. For those who have hardened veins, so that the blood cannot have its natural flow and they cannot keep down what they have eaten, take the juice of this same plant and give it to drink. Then take wine, honey, and water and mix them together; it will quicky heal the illness.
4. For liver pain, gather the same plant on Midsummer's Day and grind it into powder.[101] Then take five spoonfuls of the powder and three cupfuls of good wine, mix them together, and give this to drink. It will be of great benefit and in the same manner will benefit other discomfort.
5. For the disease in which stones develop in the bladder, take the roots of the same plant and pound them. Simmer them in hot wine and give it to drink; it heals the disease in a wonderful way, and not just

---

99. In Cockayne, the habitat of the plant, if it is included, is numbered paragraph 1, whereas De Vriend begins his paragraph numbering with the first *use* for the plant, and the opening paragraph with the information about habitat is unnumbered. De Vriend's numbering is retained here, as it is in the contents list. The manuscript does not have numbers beside any paragraphs; each new paragraph begins with a capital letter, however.

100. Even though a native name for the plant existed at the time, the translator uses the Latin term throughout this chapter.

101. Grieve notes under vervain that it must be picked before flowering and dried promptly; and, with regard to the remedy just before this one, she notes that since ancient times, the vervain plant has been bruised and worn about the neck for certain conditions. Culpepper says vervain flowers at Midsummer, which agrees well with the *Herbarium*'s advice about when to gather this plant for medicinal use.

that one: it also quickly clears away anything that prevents the flow of urine and carries it away.

6.   For headache, take the same *uermenaca* [vervain] plant and bind it on the head; it will lessen the headache.[102]

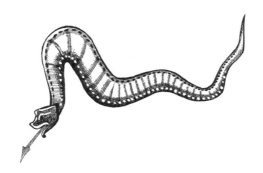

7.   For snakebite: all who have this plant with its leaves and roots on them are able to resist all snakebites.

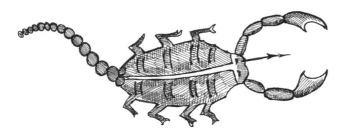

8.   For the bite of a poisonous spider, take the leaves of this same plant, simmer them, bruised, in wine. If there is a swelling where the poison is retained, lay it on there. The swelling will quickly open. After

---

102. C = For a head sore. . . . it will make to wane the sore of the head.

it has opened up, then crush the plant with honey and lay it on there until the place clears up; that will be very quickly.

9. For the bite of a mad dog, take the same plant, *uermenaca* [vervain], and whole grains of wheat.[103] Lay them on the bite so that the grains are softened by the moisture and become swollen; then take the grains and throw them to some chickens. If they refuse to eat them, then take other grains and mix with the plant in the same way as you did earlier and lay this on the bite until you feel that the danger is gone and drawn out.

10. For fresh wounds, take the same plant, mix it in butter, and lay it on the wound.

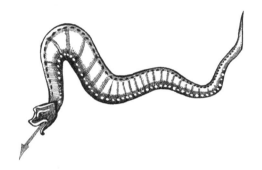

11. For snakebite, take twigs of the same plant, simmer them in wine, and then pound them. If the location of the bite cannot be seen,[104] and if the swelling has not come to a head, then lay the plant on it and it will quickly open. As soon as it opens, take the same plant, unsoaked, and crush it with honey. Lay it on the sore until it has healed; that will be very quickly if one puts it on in this way.

5. Henbane (*Hyoscyamus niger L.*), *symphoniaca, Hennebelle* or *Belone*

This plant, called *symphoniacum* and *belone* and also henbane, grows in cultivated ground, in sandy soil, and in gardens. There is another of this same plant, dark in color[105] and with stronger and poisonous leaves. The former is whiter and it has the following powers:

1. For earache, take the juice of this same plant, warm it, and drip it into the ear; it puts the earache to flight in a wonderful way. Likewise, if worms are present, it kills them.

---

103. C = wheaten corns hole.
104. C = if the scratch is blind.
105. C = swart in hue.

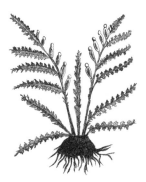

2. For swollen knees or calves or wherever on the body there is a swelling, take the same plant, *simphoniaca* [henbane], crush it, and lay it on; it will take away the swelling.
3. For toothache, take the roots of this same plant, simmer in strong wine, drink it very warm and hold in the mouth; it will quickly heal the toothache.
4. For pain or swelling of the genitals, take the roots of the same plant and fasten them to the thigh; it will make both the pain and the swelling of the genitals take flight.
5. If a woman's breasts are painful, take the juice of this same plant, make it into a drink, give it to her to drink, and smear the breasts with it; she will quickly be better.
6. For sore feet, take the same plant with its roots and pound them together; lay them on the feet and bind them on; it cures wonderfully and the swelling goes away.
7. For lung disease, take the juice of the same plant and give it to drink; the person will be remarkably cured.[106]

6. Snakeweed[107] (*Polygonum bistorta L.*), *uiperina, Nædderwyrt*

This plant, called *uiperina* or snakeweed, grows in water and in fields; it has tender leaves and is bitter to the taste.

1. For snakebite, take the same plant, *uiperina* [snakeweed], pound it, and mix it with wine. Give it to drink; it cures the bite wonderfully[108] and expels the poison. You must gather the plant in the month of April.

---

106. C = For lungs addle (disease). . . . with high wondering he will be healed.
107. Literally snakeplant (*nædre wort* in Old English); also called adderwort and viperina in modern English.
108. C = it healeth wondrously the rent.

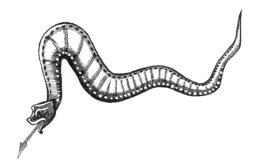

7. Sweet Flag[109] (*Acorus calamus L.*), *ueneria, Beowyrt*

This plant, which is *ueneria* in Latin and sweet flag in our language, is grown in cultivated places, in garden plots, and in meadows; you should gather the plant in the month of August.

1. So that bees do not swarm and leave, take the same plant that we call *ueneria* [sweet flag] and hang it on the hive; they will remain and will never depart, on the contrary, it will please them.[110] This plant is seldom found, and it cannot be recognized except when it grows and blooms.[111]

2. If someone cannot urinate, and the urine has stopped, take the roots of this same plant, simmer them down in water by two-thirds, and give this to drink. Within three days, the person will be able to pass urine; it cures the condition wonderfully.

8. Lion's Foot or Lady's Mantle (*Alchemilla vulgaris L.*), *pedem leonis, Leonfot*

This plant, called *pedem leonis* or lion's foot [or lady's mantle], grows in fields, in ditches, and in beds of reeds.

---

109. The Old English means literally bee plant. Bierbaumer alone identifies this plant as *Melissa officinalis L.* because of the reference to its preventing bees from swarming ("wegen der Verwendung gegen das Abschwärmen der Bienen"). Dioscorides III, 18, and Grieve also say that *Melissa* is said to delight bees. How the reference to bees originally got into the uses for this plant is not known; it is present in the Latin version as well. *Akoron* in Dioscorides I, 2 is *Iris pseudacorus* or yellow flag, a cousin to sweet flag. The illustration in Cotton Vitellius C. iii would support the majority in identifying this plant as sweet flag; a major feature of this plant, according to Grieve, is its large rhizome that grows sideways, not down, from which numerous roots grow. Grieve also mentions its sword-shaped leaves. The sideways-growing rhizome, the roots, and sword-shaped leaves are all shown in the manuscript illustration.
110. C = *ac hym gelicað*: it will like them well.
111. *blewð*: C = blows.

1. If someone has the condition of being under an evil spell, you can untie them from it:[112] Take five of the plants we call lion's foot without their roots, simmer them in water while the moon is waning, and wash the person with it. Lead the person out of the house in the early evening and fumigate him with the birthwort plant. When going outside, the person must not look back; in this way you can undo the condition.[113]

9. Celery-Leaved Crowfoot (*Ranunculus sceleratus L.*), *scelerata*, *Clufeunge*[114]

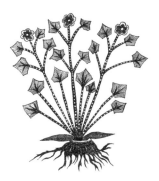

This plant, named *scelerata* or crowfoot, grows in damp and watery places; whoever eats this plant on an empty stomach will die laughing.

1. For wounds and for carbuncles, take this same plant, mix it with unsalted grease, put it onto the wound, and then eat the plant; it will cleanse if any pus is present.[115] However, do not let it stay there longer than necessary, or it will eat into healthy skin. If you want to test this as an experiment, bruise the plant and bind it onto your healthy hand; it will quickly eat into the flesh.
2. For swellings and for warts, take this same plant, mix it with pig's dung, and put it on the swelling and the wart; within a few hours it will drive out the pain and draw out the pus.

---

112. DeV explains in a note that the Latin original, *defixus*, has such a meaning; the Old English here is *sy cis*, to be under a spell. C = be choice (in eating), which is the meaning given in BT.

113. *Curanderas* still frequently prescribe remedies for *mal de ojo*, conditions caused by being looked at by someone with an evil eye. Several other ailments are caused by being put (or putting oneself) under a spell of some kind. The conditions are said to be easily recognized if one is trained to diagnose them. Birthwort (20) is twice prescribed in the *Herbarium* as a smudge stick to provide healing smoke.

114. C = clofthing or cloffing; Cockayne has the correct botanical identification but this unusual English translation.

115. *hwæt horwes on bið*. C = anything of foulness.

10. Buttercup (*Ranunculus acris L.*), *batracion, Clufwyrt*[116]

This plant, called *batracion* and also buttercup, grows in sandy soil and in fields; it has few leaves, and they are thin.

1. For a lunacy, take the plant and bind it around the person's neck with a piece of red thread when the moon is on the wane in the month of April and in early October; the person will be quickly healed.
2. For sores that have turned dark,[117] take the same plant with its roots, pound them, mix vinegar with it, and put this on the sore; it will quickly heal it and will make it like the rest of the body.

11. Mugwort (*Artemesia vulgaris L.*), *artemesia, Mucgwyrt*

This plant, called *artemesia* and also mugwort, grows in rocky and sandy places. If someone wants to begin a journey, the person should take some *artemesia* [mugwort] in hand and keep it with him; then the person won't feel the hardship of the journey too much. It also expels demonic possession. In a house where it is present, it prevents bad medications and it also turns away the evil eye.[118]

1. For soreness of the abdomen, take the same plant, make it into a powder, mix it with new beer, and give it to drink; it will quickly ease the abdominal pain.
2. For sore feet, take the same plant, mix it with grease, and put it on the feet; it takes away the soreness of the feet.

12. Mugwort/Tansy (*Tanacetum vulgaris L*), *artemesia tagantes, Mucgwyrt*[119]

1. For bladder pain and when a person cannot urinate, take the juice of this plant, which is also called mugwort (it is, however, another kind) and simmer it in hot water or in wine and give it to drink.

---

116. C = clove wort. BT has "buttercup," and this is a type of buttercup.

117. *ða sweartan dolh.* C = the swart scars.

118. Literally, this says to turn away the eyes of an evil person, but I believe it is another reference to the *mal de ojo* (evil eye). C = evil eyes of evil men. He also adds here "he, the man of the house" to explain who in the house would have the plant; the Anglo-Saxon reads literally "in the house where one has it (the plant) inside."

119. No painting appears for this plant in the Cotton manuscript, although in the contents list, *herba artemisia tagantes* (chapter 12) is listed as another kind of mugwort. Cockayne's numbering of the mugworts reflects the Latin originals, which had three separate chapters for the artemisias, a very large family of bitter plants. Dioscorides, too, lists three artemisias in a row as III, 127, 128, and 129, but they do not correspond exactly to the Old English original. That three artemisias occur together is noteworthy, and the identification may have changed over the centuries to match where the compiler lived. D'A says that André identifies this plant as *Tanacetum vulgare L.* or tansy. Bierbaumer, C, and DeV = *Artemesia dracunculus* (tarragon).

2. For soreness in the thighs, take the same plant, mix it with grease, and wash it well with vinegar; bandage it on the sore; on the third day the person will be better.
3. For sore tendons and for swelling, take the same plant, *artemesia* [mugwort], mix it with oil that has been well boiled; apply it; it heals wonderfully.
4. If someone is greatly and heavily tormented with gout, take the roots of this same plant, give to eat in honey, and soon afterward the person will be cured and cleansed in a way that that you never suspected it might have such great power.
5. If someone is afflicted with fever, take the juice of this same plant with oil and apply it; the fever will leave the person quickly.[120]

13. Wormwood (*Artemesia pontica L.*), *artemisia leptefilos, Mucgwyrt*

The third plant, which we call *artemesia leptefilos,* wormwood,[121] or mugwort, grows around ditches and in old dirt mounds; if you break off its blossoms, it has the smell of elder.

1. For stomachache, take this plant, pound it, and simmer it well in almond oil in the way in which you make a poultice. Then put it on a clean piece of cloth and lay it on the stomach; within five days the person will be well. If the roots of this plant are hung over the door of a house, then no one may do harm to the house.
2. For trembling in the tendons, take the juice of this same plant mixed with oil and rub it on there; it quiets the tremors and takes away the entire condition.

Indeed, about the three plants that we call *artemisia* [mugwort], it is said that Diana found them and gave knowledge of their power and medicinal value to the centaur Chiron, who was the first to prescribe a medicine using this plant and who named the plant *artemisia* after Diana.[122]

---

120. This is a good example of a remedy being given in shorthand for someone who would know how to interpret it. How much of the plant juice to add, whether it would be obtained by infusing the plant or other means, in what kind of oil to mix it and with how much, and where to put it on the patient would all be up to the healer, who knew by experience how to put this—and other like remedies—together, much like the shorthand cooking recipes with which most people are familiar.

121. *Artemesia pontica* is roman wormwood; *artemesia leptefilos* is southernwood (III, 128 in Dioscorides; not listed by this name in Grieve who calls southernwood *artemesia abrotanum*). D'A says that André identifies this plant as *Artemisia campestris L.* Because of the number of artemesias in any locale, the practitioner would have to learn which one was meant from one who knew the plants.

122. Recall that one of the figures named on the title page (19r) is Chiron the centaur.

14. Dock (*Rumex spp. L.*), *lapatium, Docce*

This plant, called *lapatium* or dock, grows in sandy places and on old dunghills.

1. For glandular swellings that grow in the genitals, take the *lapatium* [dock] plant and pound it in aged unsalted grease so that there are two parts more of the grease than of the plant. When it is well mixed, form it into a ball, enfold it in a cabbage leaf,[123] and let it smoke on hot ashes. When it is hot, lay it on the swellings, and fasten it there. This is best for these swellings.

15. Dragonswort (*Dracunculus vulgaris, Arum dracunculus L.*), *dracontea, Dracentse*[124]

About this plant, which is called *dracontea*[125] and also dragonswort, it is said that it should be grown in dragon's blood. It grows at the tops of mountains where there are groves of trees, chiefly in holy places and in the country that is called Apulia.[126] It grows in stony soil, it is soft to the touch and sweet like green chestnuts in taste, and the root below is like a dragon's head.

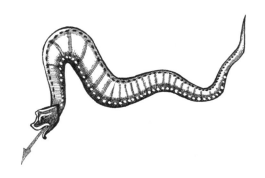

---

123. *caules leafe*, a plant described in *Herbarium* 130, where C and DeV identify it as *Brassica napus* or rape (also colewort), a type of mustard. D'A identifies it as *Brassica oleracea*, cabbage, citing Maggiulli, *Nomenclatura delle piante*, p. 173. C's translation of the leaf is cabbage.

124. C, DeV, and D'A identify this plant as *Dracunculus vulgaris* or *Arum dracunculus L.* and the plant in chapter 6, *nædre wyrt*, as *Polygonum bistorta*. Hunt identifies both as "bistort" *(Polygonum bistorta)*. Grieve says that the Arum family is enormous and that the roots are used for many purposes; her description of how arums grow is very close to the drawing in the Cotton MS.

125. C puts the plant name in Greek here; however the OE does not have it.

126. Groves of trees have been holy places from the most ancient times in many cultures; see Sir James G. Frazer, *The Golden Bough* (New York: The Macmillan Company, 1940).

1. For all snakebites, take the roots of the *dracontea* [dragonswort] plant, pound it with wine, warm it, and give it to drink. All the poison will disappear.
2. For broken bone, take the roots of this same plant and mix them with grease, just like you make a poultice. The broken bones will appear out of the body.[127]

You should gather the plant in the month called July.

16. Orchis, Wild Orchid (*Orchis spp. L.*), *satyrion, Hreafnes leac*

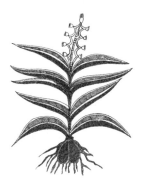

This plant, which is called *satyrion* or wild orchid,[128] grows on high mountains, in hard places, in meadows, and in cultivated and sandy lands.

1. For painful wounds,[129] take the roots of the plant we call *satyrion* [orchis] and also some call *priapiscus* and pound them together. It cleanses the wounds and soothes the pain.
2. For eye pain, that is, when one is blear-eyed, take the juice of the same plant and apply to the eyes. Without delay it takes away the pain.

---

127. Clearly a step is missing in the instructions—that of applying the medicine. Such omissions are common throughout the *Herbarium,* but in the hands of someone familiar with this type of medicine, such obvious steps would not be necessary to spell out.

128. C gives a Greek name that is not in the original. C calls this plant ravens leek, but notes that it is in the Orchis (orchid) family.

129. *earfoðliche wundela.* C = difficult wounds.

17. Yellow Gentian (*Gentiana lutea L.*), *gentiana, Feldwyrt*[130]

This plant, which is called *gentiana* and also yellow gentian, grows in the mountains and on hills. It improves all tonics.[131] It is soft to the touch and bitter to the taste.

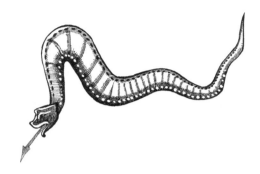

1.   For snakebite, take the root of the *gentiana* [gentian] plant, dry it, then pound it into a powder[132] weighing about four grams; give it to drink in three cups of wine. It helps a great deal.

18. Cyclamen, Sowbread (*Cyclamen europaeum L.*), *orbicularis, Slite*[133]

This plant, called *orbicularis* and also sowbread, grows in cultivated places and in hilly lands.

1.   For hair loss,[134] take the same plant and put it in the nostrils.
2.   For irritable bowels, take the same plant, make it into a salve, and put it where the abdomen is sore. It also helps heartburn.[135]
3.   For pain in the spleen, take one cup of the juice of this plant and five spoonfuls of vinegar. Give this to drink for nine days; you will be

---

130. C = field wort (*Erythraea pulcella Sw.*). Bierbaumer has Autumn Gentian (*Gentiana amarella L.*), all in the same family of plants. D'A and DeV agree on *Gentiana lutea L.*

131. *heo framað to eallum drenceom.* C = is beneficial for all drinks (antidotes). Grieve explains at length how the gentian root was used in many kinds of tonics.

132. *cnuca to duste.* C = knock it to dust.

133. C has *Cyclamen hederaefolium*, which Grieve says is very close to the species that Bierbaumer and DeV prefer. Grieve notes that the roots are a favorite food of swine, hence the name.

134. *wiþ þæt ðæt mannes fex fealle.* Literally: if the hair of a person falls out. DeV says in a note that the translator confused *deplere* with *depilare*. The Latin original DeV uses has *Ad caput deplendum.* The meaning is not appreciably different in either case.

135. *heortece.* C = heartache, a term that is not equivalent to heartburn in modern English.

surprised about its effects. Also take the roots of the same plant and hang them around a person's neck so that they hang in front against the spleen. The person will be cured quickly. Whoever drinks the juice of this plant will quickly experience wonderful relief in the abdomen.

One can collect the plant at any time of the year.

19. Knotgrass (*Polygonum aviculare L.*), *proserpinaca, Unfortrædde*[136]

This plant, called *proserpinaca* or knotgrass, grows everywhere in cultivated places and on mounds. You should pick the plant in summer.

1. If a person vomits blood, take the juice of the *proserpinaca* [knot-grass] plant and simmer it without letting it steam[137] in good, strong wine. Give it to drink on an empty stomach for nine days. In this time you will see wonderful effects from it.
2. For pain in the sides, take the juice of this same plant in oil and rub it on frequently. It will soothe the pain.
3. For a woman's sore nipples[138] when nursing and swollen, take the same plant, pound it, soften it in butter, and put it on the nipples. It will soothe the swelling and soreness wonderfully.
4. For eye pain; before the sun rises or just before it fully begins to set, go to the same plant, *proserpinaca* [knotgrass], and mark around it with a golden ring. Say that you want to pick it to make a medicine for the eyes.[139] Three days later, go again before sunrise, pick the plant, and hang it around the person's neck. It will help a great deal.
5. For earache, take the juice of this same plant made lukewarm and drip it into the ear. It chases away the pain wonderfully. And also, we have found honestly and truly ourselves that it helps. Also, it certainly heals sores on the outside of the ears.
6. For diarrhea, take the juice of the leaves of this plant and boil gently in water. Give it to drink in the quantity you think suitable, and the person will be well.

---

136. C = Untrodden to Pieces as the literal translation of the OE name of this plant.
137. *butan smice gewyl.* C = boil it without smoke. Those familiar with perparing herbal reme-dies would understand that the meaning here is not without smoke from the fire, but without the plume of vapor a liquid makes when it is boiling fast.
138. *titta sár wifa.* C = for sore of titties of women.
139. The habit of speaking to plants before picking them (with the allied caution of not picking too many of the same plant in any one locality to save the species) is a basic tenet for many who collect medicinal plants in the wild.

20. Heartwort, birthwort (*Aristolochia rotunda* or *clematis L.*), *aristolochia,*
Smerowyrt

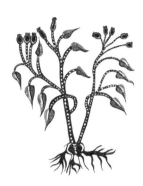

This plant, called *aristolochia* or birthwort, grows on hilly lands and in firm
places.

1.   Against the strength of poison, take the *aristolochia* [heartwort]
     plant and pound it. Give it to drink in wine, and it will overcome all
     the strength of the poison.
2.   For the most violent of fevers, take the same plant and dry it. Fumi-
     gate the person with it; it chases away not only the fever, but also
     similar demon-like illnesses.[140]
3.   For sore nostrils, take the roots of this same plant and put them in the
     nostrils; it will quickly purge them and lead to healing. In truth, heal-
     ers cannot cure much without this plant.
4.   If someone is weakened by chills, take the same plant, oil, and pig's
     grease, and mix them together. It has the strength to warm the person.
5.   For snakebite, take ten pennies' weight of the roots of the same plant
     in half a pitcher of wine.[141] Soak them together, and give it to drink
     often. It will expel the poison.

---

140. *swylce deofulseocnyssa.* The hallucinations often associated with high fevers and similar
conditions could be described in such a way. C = devil sickness or demoniacal possession.

141. The measure (*healfne sester wines*) for the amount of wine prescribed is discussed in DeV,
lxxxi–lxxxiv. A *sester* was a jug or pitcher full, which I would guess is a liter (a little more than
a quart), since this has been a customary amount of liquid for a long time. C gives three-quarters
of a pint. Also note that Grieve's description of the various Aristolochias bears out the need for
caution in using the correct amount of this plant; too much of it will cause terrible pain in the
abdomen and bowels.

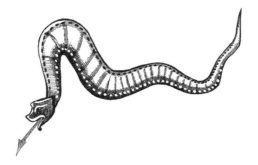

6. If a child is very upset,[142] take the same plant and fumigate the child with it. You will make it happier.
7. If anyone has a sore growing on the nose, take the same plant, cypress, dragonswort, and honey; pound them together and lay this on the sore. It will soon heal.

21. Watercress, Garden Cress (*Nasturtium officinale* or *Lepidum sativum L.*), *nasturcium, Cærse*

1. If a person's hair is falling out, take the juice of the plant that is called *nasturcium* or cress. Put it in the nose. The hair will grow.

This plant is not sown, but propagates itself in springs and in brooks. It is also written that in some countries it will grow next to walls.

2. For head sores, that is for dandruff or itching, take the seeds of this plant and goose grease, and mix them together. It draws the whiteness of the dandruff off of the head.
3. For soreness in the body, take the same *nasturcium* [cress] plant and pennyroyal and simmer them in water; give this to drink. You will improve the body's soreness, and the illness will depart.
4. For swellings, take the same plant, mix it with oil, and lay it on the swellings. Take the leaves of the same plant and lay them on also.
5. For warts, take the same plant and yeast, mix them together, lay this on the wart, and it will soon be taken away.

---

142. *ahwæned.* C = vexed. However BT gives the Latin as *vexare, contristare, molestare*, all of which connote being upset or afraid more than angry. The Latin cited by DeV is *contristus.* See also its use in item 2: Obviously the burned leaves of this plant used as a smudge helped in healing.

22. Meadow Saffron (*Colchicum autumnale L.*), *hieribulbum, Greate wyrt*[143]

This plant, called *hieribulbus* or meadow saffron, grows around hedges and in putrid places.[144]

1. For soreness in the joints, take six ounces of the plant we call *hieribulbus* [meadow saffron] the same amount of goat's grease, and one pound plus two ounces of oil from the cypress tree. Pound them together until well mixed. It relieves pain both of the insides and of the limbs.
2. If pimples grow on a woman's nose, take the roots of the same plant and mix them with oil, then wash with it. It will cleanse away all the pimples.

23. No English Name (*Witharia somnifera*), *apollinaris, Glofwyrt*[145]

About this plant, which is called *apollinaris* and also *glofwyrt*, it is said that Apollo found it first and gave it to the healer Aesculapius.[146] From that, he gave the name to it.

1. For sore hands, take the same plant, *apollinaris*, pound it with unsalted, aged grease. Add to it one cup of aged wine, and heat it without letting any steam rise (let there be one pound of the grease). Pound together as you would a poultice and smear it on the hands.

24. Camomile (*Anthemis nobilis L.*), *camemelon, Mageþe*

1. For eye pain, let the person pick the plant called *camemelon* or camomile before sunrise.[147] When picking it, the person should say he is picking it for white specks in the eye and for eye pain.[148] Then take the juice and apply it to the eyes.

---

143. Only D'A gives André's suggestion that this plant is *herba hieribulbum* (*Muscari comosum*), tassel hyacinth.

144. Perhaps dung heaps or privies is meant here, known sources of rich soil.

145. C, DeV, Bierbaumer = lily of the valley. D'A citing Maggiulli and André, identifies the plant as *herba apollinaris* (*Withania somnifera*). She says that lily of the valley appears only late in herbals and believes there is no modern name in English for the plant that is actually described here. Hunt suggests the name *apollinaris* might have been used for lily of the valley, foxglove, mandrake, and black nightshade.

146. Here is another figure named on the title page (19r).

147. As an example of C's style: For sore of eyes, let a man take ere the upgoing of the sun, the wort which is called $Xαμαίμηλον$. C supplies the Greek letters for the name although they are not in the manuscript. For some reason, C begins here often to substitute "ooze" for "juice" in his translation.

148. See note at chapter 19 about collectors' talking to plants before picking them as a matter of respect. Picking plants before the sun is hot is customary so that few volatile oils and saps are dissipated by the heat.

25. Wall Germander (*Teucrium chamaedris L.*), *chamedris, Heortclæfre*[149]

This plant, called *chamedris* or germander, grows on hills and in hard soil.

1.   If a person is bruised, take the plant we call *chamedris* [germander],
     pound it in a wooden vessel and give it to drink in wine. It also heals
     a bite or sting.

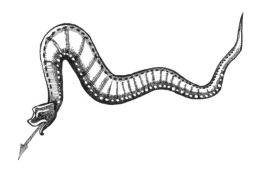

2.   For snakebite, take the same plant, pound it into a powder, and give
     to drink in aged wine. It will expel the poison thoroughly.
3.   For gout, take the same plant and give it to drink in warm wine, just
     as we said before. It relieves the pain wonderfully and brings about
     healing.

   You should pick the plant in August.

26. Wild Teasel (*Dipsacus silvestris*), *chamecælæ,Wulfes Camb*

1.   For liver sickness, take the plant called *chameaeleæ* or also teasel
     and give it to drink in wine (for fever in warm water). It has wonder-
     ful benefits.
2.   For drinking poison, take the same plant, pound it into a powder, and
     give it to drink in wine. All the poison will be expelled.
3.   For dropsy, take the same plant and the same amount of spurge (fig-
     wort), wall germander, and ground-pine, and pound them into a pow-
     der. Give this to drink in wine; five spoonfuls to young men, three
     spoonfuls to youngsters, the ill, and to women, and one to little chil-
     dren.[150] It expels the water very well through the urine.

---

149. DeV notes here that *Heort-* is probably from *heorot,* hart, because deer are said to like to eat
it. He also lists other possible identifications for this plant.
150. This is a common method used by herbalists to determine dosage, based largely on the
patient's body weight and physical condition.

27. Ground-pine (*Ajuga chamaepitys* or *Teucrium chamaepitys L.*), *chamepithys, Henep*

1. For wounds, take the plant that is called *chamepithys* or ground-pine. Pound it and lay it on the wound. If the wound is deep, take the juice and wring it onto the wound.
2. For pain in the abdomen, take the same plant and give it to drink. It alleviates the pain.

28. Spurge or figwort (*Dafne L.* or *Ranunculus ficaria L.*), *chamedafne, Hræfnes fot*

1. For constipation, take the plant the Greeks call *chamedafne* and the English call spurge or figwort, pound into fine powder, and give it to drink in warm water. It stimulates the bowels.

29. Madder (*Rubia tinctorum L.*), *ostriago, Lyvwort*[151]

This plant, called *ostriago* or madder, grows around graveyards, on mounds, and on the walls of houses that stand against hills.

1. For all soreness that afflicts people, take the plant we call *ostriago* [madder], pound it, and lay it on the sore. As we said earlier, it will completely heal every painful thing that develops on the body.

If you want to pick this plant, you should be pure, and you should pick it before sunrise in the month of July.

30. Great Water Dock (*Rumex hydrolapathum L.* or *aquaticus L.*), brittanica, Heawenhnydelu[152]

1. For mouth sores, take the plant that the Greeks call *brittanice* and the English call great water dock, pound it when green, and press out the juice. Give it to drink and to hold in the mouth. Even if some of it is swallowed, it will still help.

---

151. DeV, Bierbaumer = wayfaring-tree (*Viburnum lantana L.*), which D'A says, citing Grieve, is never used for medicinal purposes. DeV says in his note to this entry that the plant is difficult to identify. C identifies it as *Sambucus ebulus.*
152. C identifies it as *Cochlearia anglica* and calls it "bright-coloured hydele." DeV notes that modern authorities identify this as the plant Pliny and Dioscorides claim cured the Roman soldiers of scurvy in the Rhine country.

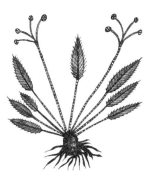

2. Again, for mouth sores, take the same plant, *brittanica* [great water dock]. If you do not have it fresh, take it dry and mix with wine to the thickness of honey. Take in the same way as we said earlier; it will have the same healing effects.
3. For toothache and if teeth are loose, take the same plant. It helps using some wonderful power. Save its juice and powdered leaves over winter because it does not grow at all times of the year. You should keep the juice in a ram's horn. Dry the powdered leaves and keep them. Moreover, taken with wine, it also helps very well for the same uses.
4. For constipation, to stimulate the bowels, take the juice of the same plant, and give it to drink undiluted, as much as the person can tolerate.[153] Without danger, it will purge the bowels.
5. For pain in the side, which the Greeks call *paralisis*, take the same plant fresh with its roots. Pound it and give two or three cupfuls to drink in wine. It is believed that it heals wonderfully.

31. Wild lettuce (*Lactuca scariola L.*), *lactuca, Wudulectric*

This plant, which is called *lactuca silfatica* or prickly lettuce, grows in cultivated and sandy soil.

1. For dimness of the eyes, it is said that when the eagle wants to fly, it will touch and wet its eyes with the juice so that it can see better, and because of that, the eagle obtains the greatest clearness.

---

153. *syle drincan be þære mihte þe hwa mæge þurch hit self.* C = give it to drink by the might, which each one may (according to a man's strength), through itself without danger . . .

2. Again, for dimness of eyesight, take the juice of the plant we call *lactuca silfatica* [wild lettuce] mixed with aged wine and honey, and this collected without smoke.[154] It is best that the juice of this plant, as we said before, be mixed with wine and honey and placed in a glass container for when it is needed. From this, you will observe a remarkable remedy.

32. Agrimony (Agrimonia eupatoria), agromonia, Garclife

1. For sore eyes, take the plant called *agrimonia* and also agrimony. Pound it fresh by itself. If you do not have it fresh, take it dried and dip it in warm water so that you can crush it easily. Apply it, and quickly it will take away the defect and the soreness from the eyes.
2. For a sore abdomen, take the root of the same plant we call *agrimonia* [agrimony], and give it to drink. It helps in a wonderful way.
3. For ulcerous sores and wounds, pick the fresh plant, bruise it, and lay it on the sore. It will cure the disorder agreeably. If you have the dried plant, dip it in warm water; it is believed that it will heal equally.

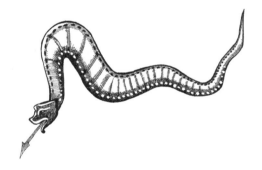

4. For snakebite, take about nine grams of the same plant and two cups of wine. Give this to drink; it expels the poison in a wonderful way.
5. For warts, take the same plant and pound it in vinegar. Lay it on, and it will make the warts disappear.
6. For soreness of the spleen, take the same plant, and give it to drink in wine. It will take away the soreness from the spleen.

---

154. Why the plant is collected without smoke remains a mystery at this point.

7. If you want to cut anything from the body, and it seems to you that you cannot, take the same plant, bruised, lay it on, and the place will open up and be healed.
8. For a blow from an iron or wooden stake, this same plant, bruised and laid on the wound, will heal it in a wonderful manner.

33. King's Spear, Asphodel (*Asphodelus ramosus L.*), *astularegia, Wudurofe*

1. For pain in the shanks of the legs or in the feet, take the juice of this plant, which is called *asphodel* or king's spear, with almond oil and rub onto where it is sore; wonderful relief will ensue. If there is swelling, pound the plant well and lay it on the sore place.
2. For pain in the liver, take the root of this same plant and give it to drink in sweetened water; it will remove the pain in a wonderful manner.

34. Dock (*Rumex L.*), *lapatium, Wududocce*

1. If any part of the body becomes stiff, take the plant that is called *lapatium* or dock, some aged pig's grease, and crumbs from oven-baked bread. Pound this together in the manner you would make a poultice, lay it on the sore place, and it helps wonderfully.

35. No English Name (*Centaurea centaurium L.*), *centauria maior, Eoregealla* or *Curmelle seo mare*[155]

1. For liver disease, take the plant that the Greeks call *centauria maior*[156] and the English used to call *curmelle seo mare* [greater centuary], simmer it in wine, and give it to drink. It strengthens the liver in a wonderful manner. Do the same for pain in the spleen.
2. For wounds and ulcerous sores, take the same plant, bruise it, and lay it on the sore. It does not allow the sore to spread.
3. This same plant, *centauria*, works very well in healing new and wide wounds so that the wounds quickly close. It also helps the flesh to knit together if one soaks the wound in water containing the plant.

---

155. C, DeV, Bierbaumer = yellow centaury. Grieve discusses several types of centaury plants, but groups them under *Erythraea centarium,* which Hunt does as well. According the Grieve, many varieties grew throughout Europe, all with similar healing properties. This does seem to be some kind of centaury plant. The third synonym in the original for the plant is *eorþgealle;* I obtained "yellow wort" from Hunt's entry under *Centaurea.*

156. Because there is no modern English name for this particular kind of centaury plant, according to D'Aronco and Cameron, an additional name given in the Old English original, *7 eac sumne men eorðgeallan hatað* (some call "earth-gall") has been omitted here (but see note 155).

36. Common or Lesser Centaury (*Centaurium umbellatum*), *centauria minor, Feferfuge, Curmelle seo læsse*

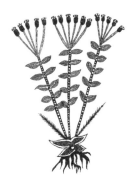

This plant, which is called *centauria minor* or lesser centaury, and which some call feverwort, grows in solid and sandy earth. It is also said that Chiron the Centaur found the plants that we call greater and lesser centaury, from which they have the name "centauries."[157]

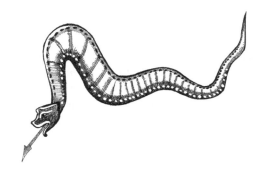

1. For snakebite, take this plant in powdered form, or the plant itself bruised, and give it to drink in aged wine; it will cure quickly.
2. For eye pain, take the juice of this same plant and apply it to the eyes; it helps poor vision. In addition, mix some honey with it, and it will certainly help dim eyesight, so that sharpness of vision will be restored.

---

157. Chiron is a figure shown on the title page 19r.

3. If anyone is dangerously ill,[158] take a good handful of this plant and
    simmer it in wine or in ale so that there is a jug full of wine. Let it
    stand for three days. Then take a half a jug full every day as needed
    mixed with honey. Drink this on an empty stomach.
4. For nerve spasms,[159] take the same plant, simmer it down in water by
    two-thirds. Give this to drink as much as the person wants and needs
    to; the person will be healed.
5. If poison has been ingested, take the same plant, pound it in vinegar,
    and give it to drink; it will quickly eliminate the poison. Also, take
    ten pennies' weight of the roots of this plant, put it in wine, and give
    three cupfuls to drink.
6. In case worms irritate the area around the anus, do as we indicated
    before for nerve spasms, that is you take the same plant and simmer
    down in water by two-thirds; it will drive the worms out.

37. Burdock (*Arctium lappa L.*), *personacia, Boete*[160]

1. For all wounds and for snakebite, take the juice of this plant, which is
    called *personacia* or burdock, and give it to drink in aged wine. It
    cures all snakebites in a wonderful way.
2. For fevers, take the leaves of this same plant and bind them on the
    feverish person. The fever will quickly disappear.
3. If a cancer sore grows on a wound, take the plant, boil it gently in
    water, and bathe the wound with it. Then take the plant, soap, and
    grease; pound them in vinegar. Put this on a cloth and lay it on the
    wound.
4. For pain in the abdomen, take one cup of the juice of the same plant
    and two cups of honey. Give this to drink on an empty stomach.
5. For the bite of a mad dog, take the roots of this same plant, pound
    them with coarse salt, and lay this on the bite.
6. For fresh wounds that are still wet,[161] take equal amounts of the the
    roots of the same plant and hawthorn leaves. Pound them together
    and lay this on the wounds.

---

158. *gyf hwa þonne on þas frecnysse befealle.* C = if anyone then fall into this mischief. Centaury was widely used for fever, according to Grieve. It would seem logical that the danger (not
mischief) here is a medical condition, perhaps from fever, from being ill, or having physical
symptoms caused by a spell such as *mal de ojo*. The Latin original in DeV does not say why this
is prescribed, but simply gives the remedy.
159. C translates the Old English term as spasm of sinews, but BT and DeV also translate *sinu*
(*seonu*) as nerve, sinew or tendon.
160. C, DeV = beet (with doubts) D'A notes that the identification of *personacia* with beet may
be due to the illustration. Hunt says personacia is a name given to large-leaved plants including
burdock, beet, and water lily.
161. *wið niwe wunda þa þe þone wætan gewyrceaþ.* C = for new wounds which work up the wet
or humour.

38. Wild Strawberry (*Fragaria vesca*), *fraga, Streawberge*

This plant, which is called *fraga* or wild strawberry, grows in shady places, in cultivated spots, and on hills.

1. For pain of the spleen, take the juice of the same plant we call wild strawberry and honey. Give it to drink, and it will help in a wonderful way.
2. The juice of this same plant taken mixed with honey and pepper helps many who have asthma or abdominal pain.

39. Marshmallow (*Althaea officinalis L.*), *Hibiscus, Merscmealuwe*

This plant, called *hibiscus* or marshmallow, grows in damp places and in fields.

1. For gout, take the plant we call *hibiscus* [marshmallow] and pound it with aged lard. Lay this on the painful spot, and in three days it will be healed. Many authorities attest to the efficacy of this plant.
2. For any accumulation of diseased matter on the body, take the same plant, simmer with fenugreek,[162] linseed, and flour. Lay it on the sore, and it will banish all the hardness.

40. Horsetail (*Equisetum L.*), *ippirus*, no OE word

1. If a person has a swollen stomach, take the juice of the plant the Greeks call *ippirus* and the Romans *æquiseia* in sweetened wine and give two cups of it to drink. It is firmly believed that it helps the condition.
2. If anyone coughs up blood, take the juice of this same plant, simmer in strong wine without letting vapors rise, and drink it on an empty stomach. It will quickly staunch the blood.

41. Mallow (*Malva silvestris L.*), *malua eratica, Hocleaf*

This plant, which is called *malua eratica* and also common mallow, grows everywhere in cultivated locations.

1. For bladder pain, take one pound of the plant that we call *malua eratica* [mallow] with its roots, simmer it down in water by one half or until the water measures two cupfuls or more. It should be simmered down within three days, as we said before, by half.[163] Give it to drink on an empty stomach; it will cure the patient.

162. *wyllecærse.* C = cress (which he says is *trigonella* in Latin, but that is fenugreek).
163. *7 þæt sy binnan þrim dagum gewylled, swa we ær cwædon, to healfan dæle.* C = let that be boiled within three days, as we said before, to a half part.

2. For sore tendons, take the same plant, pound it with aged grease. It soothes the tendons wonderfully.
3. For a pain in the side, take the same plant, simmer it in ale, and after you have simmered it, place it in a mortar together with its leaves and pound it. Put it in a cloth and lay it onto the side, and do not take it off for three days. You will alleviate the pain.
4. For fresh wounds, take the roots of this same plant and burn them into powder,[164] then put this onto the wound.

42. Alkanet *(Anchusa officinalis L.), buglossa, Hundes Tunge, (Glofwyrt)*[165]

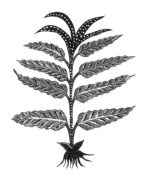

This plant, which the Greeks call *buglossa* and the Romans *lingua bubula* and the English alkanet, grows in cultivated places and in sandy soil.

1. If anyone has tertian or quartan fever, take the roots of this plant when the plant has three pods of seeds. Simmer the roots in water and give it to drink; you will cure the person.

Plants that have four pods of seeds cure exactly the same as we said earlier.

Another plant is similar to this one; it has somewhat smaller leaves than dock; its roots taken in water act against toads and snakes.

2. For asthma or shortness of breath, take the same plant, honey, and bread that has been baked using grease, just like you make a poultice. It takes away the pain in a wonderful way.

---

164. Possibly roasted in the oven or over a fire and then ground into a powder.
165. C, DeV, Bierbaumer = bugloss or hound's-tongue (*Cynoglossum officinale L.*) All question its actual identity. DeV says that *glofwyrt* is an erroneous synonym for *hundes tunge.*

43. Sea Onion, Squill (*Scilla maritima L.* or *Urgina maritima*),
bulbiscillitica,Glædene

1. For dropsy, take the plant called *bulbiscillitici* or squill, and dry it
    completely. Take the inner part of the plant and simmer it in water.
    When it is warm, mix with it honey and vinegar. Give three cupfuls,
    and quickly the sickness will be drawn out through the urine.
2. For painful joints, take the same plant, as we said earlier, the inside
    part, and simmer it in ale. Rub the sore place with this and it will heal
    quickly.
3. For the condition the Greeks call *paronichias* [chilblains], take the
    roots of this same plant, pound them with vinegar and some bread,
    and then lay it on the sore. It cures the condition in a wonderful way.
4. For thirst that cannot be quenched when suffering from dropsy, take
    a leaf from this same plant and put it under the tongue. Soon the
    thirst will be prevented.

44. Navelwort (*Cotyledon umbilicus*), *cotiledon*, no OE word

This plant, which the Greeks call *cotiledon* and the Romans *umbilicum
uereris*, grows on roofs and on mounds.

1. For swellings, take this plant and pig's grease (however, for women,
    unsalted) each in equal amounts by weight and pound them together.
    Put this on the swelling, and it will disappear. You should pick the
    plant in wintertime.

45. Cockspur grass (*Panicum crus galli*), *gallicrus*, *Attorlaðe*

This plant, called *gallicrus* and also cockspur grass, grows in firm soil and
along roadways.

1. For dog bite, take the plant and pound it with grease and bread baked
    on the hearth. Lay this on the bite, and it will quickly be healed. This
    also helps cure hard swellings, and it removes them.

46. Horehound (*Marrubium vulgare*), *prassion*, *Harehune*

1. For a cold in the head and for heavy coughing, take the plant the
    Greeks call *prassion,* the Romans *marubium,* and the English hore-
    hound, and simmer it in water. Give it to drink whenever the cough-
    ing is heavy, and it will help wonderfully.
2. For a stomachache, take the juice of this same plant and give it to
    drink. It takes away a stomachache. If fever bothers the person, give
    the same plant well diluted in water, and it will restore health.

3. For worms around the anus, take equal amounts by weight of the *maribium* [horehound] plant, wormwood, and lupin, and simmer them two or three times in sweetened water and wine. Put this on the anus, and it will kill the worms.

4. For painful and swollen joints, take the same plant, burn it to ashes, put it on the sore, and it will quickly heal.

5. If someone tastes poison, take the juice of this plant, simmer it in aged wine, and drink it. Quickly it will be better.

6. For scabs and impetigo,[166] take the same plant, simmer it in water, and wash the body with it where there are sores. It removes the scabs and the impetigo.

7. For lung disease, take the same plant and simmer it in honey. Give it to eat, and the person will be cured in a wonderful manner.

8. For all stiffness in the body, take the same plant and pound it well with grease. Put this on the soreness, and it will cure it in a wonderful way.

47. Gladiolus (*Gladiolus segetum*), *xifion, Foxes fot*[167]

1. For strange carbuncles that are growing on the body, take three ounces of the root of this plant, which is called *xifion* or gladiolus, six ounces of fine flour, two cups of vinegar and three ounces of fox's grease. Pound together with wine, daub a cloth with it, lay it on the sore, and you will be amazed at the medicine.

2. For a fractured skull, take the upper part of the same plant, dry it, and pound it. Then take the same amount by weight of wine, mix them together, lay it on the sore, and it will pull the broken bone out. Also, if anything on the body is injured, it will heal that, or if anyone steps on something poisonous, a deadly snake or on an adder, with his feet. This same plant works very well against poison.

48. True Maidenhair (*Adiantum capillus-Veneris L.*), *gallitricus, Wæterwyrt*[168]

1. If swellings bother a maiden, take the plant called *gallitricus* or true maidenhair, pound it by itself, lay it on the swelling, and it will heal it.

2. If someone's hair is falling out, take the same plant, mix it with oil, rub it on the hair, and it will soon be fast.

---

166. *teter.* C = tetter. DeV = ringworm as the meaning of *teter.*
167. C, DeV = unbranched bur reed *(Sparganium emersum).*
168. C, DeV, Bierbaumer = *Callitriche verna L.,* water starwort, but D'A says this plant never appears in the herbals as a healing plant.

49. Garlic (Allium nigrum L.), temolus, Syngrene[169]

This plant is called *temolus* or garlic: Homer said it was the most splendid and that Mercury discovered it. The juice of this plant is extremely beneficial, and its root is round and dark, and also the same size as the leek.

   1.   For pain of the womb, take this plant, pound it, and lay it on; it relieves the pain.

50. Heliotrope (Heliotropium europaeum L.), æliotropus, Sigelhweorfa[170]

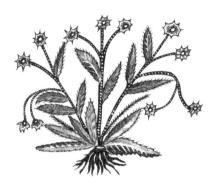

This plant, which the Greeks call *æliotrophus*, the Romans *uertamnus*, and the English heliotrope, grows everywhere in cultivated, cleared soil and in meadows.[171] The plant has some wonderful, divine properties, namely, its blossoms turn to follow the sun's course, so that when the sun sets, they close themselves, and when it rises, they open and spread themselves wide. The plant helps in the following remedies that we have written down.

   1.   For all poisons, take the same plant and pound it into fine powder, or give its juice to drink in good wine. It is a wonderful antidote to the poison.
   2.   For flux, take the leaves of this same plant, pound them, and lay them on the soreness. It is believed that it helps very effectively.

---

169. D'A notes that tradition says this is the plant Mercury gave Ulysses to escape from Circe, and it is thought to be a kind of garlic with a yellow flower (she cites Grieve, André, and Maggiulli for the identification). DeV identifies it as butterwort *(Pinguicola vulgaris L.)* and Cockayne as houseleek *(Sempervivum tectorum)*.
170. DeV and Bierbaumer say this is cat's-ear *(Hypochoeris glabra L.)*. Both reject C's identification of the plant as *Achillea tomentosa*.
171. As DeV notes, this sentence is difficult to read because of damage to the manuscript. Spellings are based on his reconstruction.

51. Madder (*Rubia tinctorum L.*), *gryas, Mæddre*

This plant, which is called *gryas* or madder and was first grown in Lucania, has the color of white marble and is adorned with four red stalks.

    1.   For aching or broken legs, take the same plant, pound it, and lay it on the leg. In three days, the place on which the poultice was laid will be much better.

    2.   Also, the roots of this same plant help heal any pain that afflicts the body; that is, when one pounds the roots and lays them on the painful place, it will heal all the soreness.

52. Common maidenhair (*Asplenium trichomanes L.*), *politricus, Hymele*[172]

This plant, called *politricus* or common maidenhair, grows on old ruins[173] and also in moist places.

    1.   For abdominal pain, take the leaves of this plant we call *politricus* [common maidenhair]—its twigs are like the bristles on a pig— pound the leaves together with nine peppercorns and nine coriander seeds. Give this to drink in good wine just before taking a bath. Also this plant is effective in making either a man's or woman's hair grow.

53. Asphodel (*Asphodelus supp. L.*), *malochin agria,Wuduhrofe*[174]

    1.   For a swollen stomach, take the roots of this plant, which the Greeks call *malochin agria*, the Romans *astula regia*, and the English asphodel, and pound them with wine. Give this to drink, and the fullness will soon go away.

    2.   For abdominal flux, take the same plant we call *astula regia* [asphodel] mixed with strong vinegar. Give this to drink, and it will bind the insides.

54. White Poppy (*Papaver somniferum L.), metoria, (Hwit) Popig*

    1.   For eye pain, which we call being blear-eyed, take the juice of the plant that the Greeks call *moecorias*, the Romans *papaver album*, and the English white poppy, or the stem of the plant with the fruit, and lay it on the eyes.

    2.   For pain at the temples of the head or headache, take the juice of this same plant, pound it with vinegar, put it on the face, and it will relieve the pain.

---

172. C, DeV = Yellow clover (*Trifolium procumbens L.*).
173. *on ealdum husstedum.* C = in old house-steads (tofts).
174. D'A following Maggiulli gives this identification. C = woodruff (*Asphodelus ramosus L.*); DeV and Bierbaumer = sweet woodruff (*Aspherula odorata*).

3.   For sleeplessness, take the juice of the same plant, rub it on the person, and you will quickly give him sleep.

55. Dropwort *(Spiraea filipendula L.)*, *oenantes, no OE word*[175]

1.   If a person cannot urinate, take the powdered roots of this plant, which is called *oennantes* or . . . [dropwort], give it to drink in two cupfuls of wine. It helps remarkably.
2.   For very bad coughs, take the roots of this same plant; take exactly as we said earlier. It relieves the coughing.

56. Narcissus or throatwort or nettle-leaved belleflower *(Narcissus poeticus L.)*, *narcisus, Halswyrt*[176]

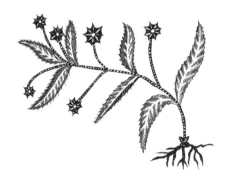

1.   For sores that grow on a person, take the roots of the plant that is called *narcisus* or narcissus pounded with oil and with flour just as you would make a poultice. Lay this on the sore, and it will heal wonderfully.

57. Spleenwort or Figwort *(Ceterach officinarum* or *Scrofularia nodosa* or *aquatica)*, *splenion, Brunewyrt*[177]

1.   For pain in the spleen, take the roots of the plant the Greeks call *splenion*, the Romans *teucerion*, and the English spleenwort, pound them into a fine powder and give this to drink in a light wine. You will

175. C, DeV = dropwort, but *Oenanthe pimpinellifolia,* not *Spiraea filipendula.*

176. C, Bierbaumer = narcissus but *Campanula trachelium L.*

177. A number of different suggestions have been made about the identification of this plant. D'A gives the meaning listed in the heading. C says it is either of the *Scrofularias* mentioned. DeV and Bierbaumer give *Asplenium ceterach L.* or *Phyllitis scolopendrium L.* D'A notes that *brunewyrt* generally denotes a fern.

experience something remarkable with it. In addition, it is said that the plant was discovered in this way: it happened that someone threw[178] some intestines, including the spleen, on this plant. The spleen quickly adhered to the plant, and the plant immediately took in the spleen, and because of this, some people called it *splenion*— spleenwort in our language. For that reason, people say about pigs, which eat the roots, that they do not have spleens.

Some also say that it has a stalk with branches like hyssop and leaves like beans, and some people call this hyssop for that reason. Gather this plant when it is in full bloom. It is famous chiefly in the mountainous lands named Cilicia and Pisidia.

58. Sage-leaved germander, wood sage, halwort, cat-thyme, polygermander (*Teucrium scorodonia* or *polium L.*), *polion*, no OE word

This plant called *polion* or . . . [germander] grows in rough places.

For insanity, take the juice of the plant we call *polion* [sage-leaved germander], mix it with vinegar, and rub it on the person who is afflicted with the evil condition before it attacks them. Put its leaves and roots in a clean cloth and fasten this around the neck of the person who suffers from the ailment; it proves itself effective.

59. Butcher's-Broom or Knee-Holly (*Ruscus aculeatus L.*), *uictoriola*, *Cneowholen*

1. For gout[179] and for the stomach, take two cups of the juice of this plant, which is called *uictoriala* or knee-holly, and give to drink on an empty stomach mixed with honey. It will quickly reduce the gout.

60. Comfrey (*Symphytum officinale L.*), *confirma*, *Galluc*

This plant, called *confirma* or comfrey, grows on the moors, in fields, and in meadows.

1. For a woman's menses,[180] take the *confirma* [comfrey] plant, pound it into fine powder, and give it to drink in wine. The flow will quickly stop.
2. If someone has an internal rupture, take the roots of this same plant and roast them in hot ashes, eat this on an empty stomach with some honey. The patient will be healed and also it completely cleans out the stomach.

178. *uppan þas wyrte gewearp.* C = scraped intestines with this plant.
179. *wiþ dropan.* C = the wrist drop. DOE, DeV = gout.
180. *wiþ wifa flewsan.* Heavy or prolonged flow is implied, or it would not need to be stopped.

3.   For stomachache, take the same plant and mix it with honey and vinegar. You will experience greatly beneficial effects.

61. Aster (*Aster amellus L.*), *asterion*, no OE word

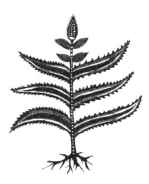

This plant, called *asterion* or . . . [aster], grows between stones and in rough places.

  This plant shines at night like the stars in the skies, and those who see it without knowing that, say they have seen an apparition, and, thus frightened, they are ridiculed by shepherds and those who know more about the power of the plant.[181]

1.   For epilepsy, take the berries of this plant that we call *asterion* [aster] and give them to eat when the moon is waning and when the sun is in the sign of Virgo, which is in the month of August. Hang the same plant around the neck. The person will be cured.

62. Hare's-Foot Clover (*Trifolium arvense L.*), *leporis pes, Haran Hyge*

1.   For constipation, take the plant that is called *leporis pes* or hare's-foot clover, dry it, make it into a powder, and give it to drink in wine if the person does not have a fever. If the person has a fever, give it to drink in water. The constipation will quickly be dispelled.

63. White Dittany or Dittany of Crete (*Dictamnus albus L.*, *origanum dictamus L.*), *dictamnus*, no OE word

This plant, which is called *dictamnus* or . . . [dittany], grows on the island named Crete and on the mountain named Ida.

---

181. C, DeV = chickweed *(Stellaria media)*. D'A = aster, because she says that chickweed does not grow on stony ground; however, Grieve says it grows virtually everywhere and also notes that chickweed flowers open about nine A.M. and are said to remain open for twelve hours, thus, into the night.

1. If a woman is carrying a dead foetus, take the juice of the plant we call *dictamnus* [dittany], and if she does not have a fever, give it to drink in wine. If she suffers from fever, give it to drink in warm water. Quickly it will purge the dead foetus without danger.

2. Again, for wounds, whether caused by iron or a pole or from a snake, take the juice of this plant and put it on the wound and give it to drink.[182] Soon the person will be well.

3. Again, for snakebite, take the juice of this plant and give it to drink in wine. It will quickly drive out the poison.

4. If anyone ingests poison, take the juice of this same plant and drink it in wine. In fact, this plant is so powerful that not only does it kill snakes with its power but also any that are near it, because of the smell. When the wind spreads the smell, wherever snakes are and smell the plant's odor, they are said to die.

It is also said about this same plant that if a ram or roe is hurt by an arrow or other weapon during a hunt, they want to eat the plant as soon as they come upon it, and that it quickly ejects the arrow and heals the wound.

5. For fresh wounds, take the same plant with stichwort and water hemp, pound them with butter, and lay this on the wound. You will be amazed at all the things this plant benefits.

64. Heliotrope (*Heliotropium spp. L.*), *solago maior*, no OE name[183]

1. For snakebite and for scorpion's sting, take the plant that is called *solago maior* and *helioscorpion* [heliotrope], dry it, and then pound it into a fine powder. Give it to drink in wine, and take the pounded plant and put it on the wound.

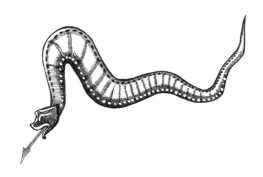

---

182. See Gross, "Schlangenliste" cited earlier.
183. C = white heliotrope. DeV = marigold.

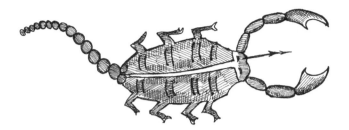

65. No English Name *(Chrosophora tinctoria Juss.), solago minor*, no OE name[184]

    1.   If worms irritate the area around the anus, take the plant that is called *solago minor* and also *æliotropion* in a dried form, make it into a fine powder and give it to drink in warm water. It will kill the worms.

66. Peony *(Paeonia officinalis L.), peonia, Peonia*

This plant, which is called *peonia* [peony], was discovered by Prince Peonius, and it gets its name from him. It grows principally in Greece, as the famous authority Homer records in his books. It is found mainly by shepherds, it has seeds the size of *maligranati*, and it shines at night like a lantern. Also, its seed is like *coccele*[185] and it is as we said earlier, most often found and gathered at night by shepherds.

    1.   For lunacy:[186] if one lays the peony plant over an insane person when he is lying down, he will quickly raise himself up healthy, and if the person has it with him, the illness will never again come near.
    2.   For sciatica, take some parts of the roots of this plant and tie them onto the sore place with a clean linen cloth. This will cure it.

---

184. C, DeV = Croton *(Croton tinctoria).*
185. DOE = cockle. DeV notes that *coccele* is a mistranslation of *granum cocci* or cochineal grain. He does not give a meaning for *maligranati,* which is pomegranate.
186. Although insanity has largely replaced lunacy (from the French word for moon) as a term for a medical condition, lunacy captures the medieval concept of what was thought to cause that condition. The moon was believed to cause "lunacy," and the Old English word for it is "month-sickness," months being measured in moons.

67. Vervain or Gipsy-Wort (*Verbena officinalis* or *Lycopus europaeus*), *peristereon, Berbene*[187]

This plant, called *peristereon* or vervain, is so much like the color of doves that some people also call it *columbina.*[188]

1. If anyone has the plant with him that we call *peristereon* [vervain], dogs will not bark at him.
2. For all kinds of poisons, take this plant powdered, give it to drink, and it will drive away the poison. It is also said that sorcerers use it for their crafts.

68. Bryony (*Bryonia L.*), *bryonia, Hymele*[189]

1. For pain in the spleen, take the plant that is called *brionia* or bryony and give it to eat mixed in food. The pain will be dispelled through urinating. This plant is agreeable enough that one can mix it with what one customarily drinks.

69. White Water Lily (*Nymfaea alba L.*), *Nimpheta,* no OE word

1a. For a swollen stomach, take the seeds of this plant, which is called *nymfeta* or . . . [white water lily], pound them with wine, and give this to drink.
1b. For the same, use the roots and give this to the patient to eat for ten days.
2. Also, if you give the plant to drink in strong wine, it stops diarrhea.[190]

70. Thistle (*Carduus supp. L.*), *crision, Claefre*[191]

1. For sore throat: If anyone has the root of the plant that is called crision or thistle and wears it tied about his neck, his throat will never trouble him.

---

187. D'A lists both of these as possibilities, but rejects DeV's suggestion that it is columbine *(Aquilegia vulgaris L.).* C and Bierbaumer proposed vervain, André Gipsy wort.
188. C notes here that the author meant columbine *(aquilegia vulgaris)* in this reference because of the color of the plant.
189. C = *Hummulus lupus* or hops.
190. *heo þæs innoðes unryne gewrið.* C = it restrains ill running *(diarrhea)* of the inwards.
191. C, DeV, and Bierbaumer = clover *(Trifolium pratense L.).* D'A says it is a type of thistle with soft spines. The manuscript drawing does not look like clover (with its distinctive three leaves).

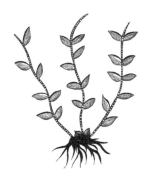

71. Woad (*Isatis tinctoria L.*), *isatis*, *Wad*

The Greeks call this plant *isatis*, the Romans *aluta*, and the English *ad serpentis morsum*.[192]

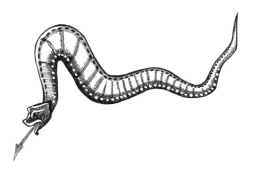

1. For snakebite, take the leaves of the plant the Greeks call *isatis* [woad] and pound them with water. Lay them on the bite. It will heal and the sore will disappear.

72. Water Germander (*Teucrium scordium L.*), *scordea*, no OE word

1. For snakebite, take the plant that is called *scordea* or . . . [water germander] and simmer it in wine. Give it to drink. Then mash the plant and lay it on the wound.

---

192. C and DeV call attention to the fact that whoever made the translation did not put the English name for woad here, but apparently by mistake copied the Latin for the next line, which reads, "for snakebite," which is the meaning of the Latin phrase. But DeV also points out the interesting fact that the same mistake occurs in MSS B and H.

2. For soreness in the joints, take the same plant, pound it, and gently boil it with the oil from a laurel tree. It will alleviate the pain.

3. For intermittent or for tertian fever, take the same plant and fasten it on the person's body. It takes away both kinds of fever.

73. Great Mullein (*Verbascum thapsus L.*), *Uerbascus, Feltwyrt*[193]

This plant, called *uerbascus* or great mullein, grows in sandy soils and on dunghills. Concerning this plant, it is said that Mercury gave it to Lord Ulysses when he met Circe, and because of it he did not fear any of her evil deeds.

1. If anyone carries with him even one twig of this plant, no terror will frighten him, no wild beast will scare him, nor will any evil approach him.[194]

2. For gout, take this same plant, *uerbascus* [great mullein], bruised. Lay it on the sore place. In a few hours, the soreness will heal to the point that the patient will dare to and be able to walk. In addition, our mentors declared and said that this preparation benefits most remarkably.

74. Herba Heraclea (*Sideritis romana L.*), *heraclea*, no OE name[195]

1. Anyone who wants to travel a long way and takes the plant called *heraclea* [herba heraclea] with him on the trip does not have to fear any robbers, for it puts them to flight.

75. Greater Celandine (*Chelidonuim maius*), *caelidonia, Cyleeenie*

1. For dimness, pain, and film in the eyes, take the juice of this plant that is called *celidonia* or greater celandine, and take the roots pounded with aged wine, honey, and pepper. When it is thoroughly mixed, apply to the inner corners of the eyes.

Also we found out that some people applied the milk of this plant to their eyes, and it helped them.

---

193. The Anglo-Saxon translator may have made a mistake in calling this plant *feldwyrt* (yellow gentian), which is the plant in chapter 17, as DeV points out in a note. The manuscript illustration looks like mullein.

194. This is one of several references to preventing or curing the condition that is thought by the *curanderas* to be caused by *mal de ojo*, evil eye.

195. C does not even name this plant, the drawing for which he deems "fantastic." DeV identifies it as *Centaurea calcitrapa L.*, star thistle, based on a gloss in MS Bodley 130, which C mentions but rejects because of the drawing in the Cotton MS. The identification used here is from D'A, who accepts André's identification, based on the Latin name for the plant, *herba heraclea*.

2. Also, for dimness of the eyes, take the juice of this same plant, or the
    blossoms pressed [of their juice] mixed with honey. Mix gently boil-
    ing ashes with this, and simmer together in a brass pot. That is a rem-
    edy exclusively for dimness of the eyes.

It is also certain that some people use just the juice, as we said earlier.

3. For swollen glands, take the same plant, pound it with lard, and lay it
    on the swelling; bathe the swelling first with water.
4. For headache, take the same plant, pound it with vinegar, and rub it
    on the face and the head.
5. For burns, take the same plant, pound it with goat's grease, and lay it
    on the burn.

76. Black Nightshade (*Solanum nigrum L.*), *solata*, *Solsequia*[196]

1. For swellings, take this plant that is called *solata* or black nightshade
    pounded and mixed with oil. Lay it on the swelling, and it will heal.
2. For earache, take the juice of this same plant, mix it with cypress
    oil,[197] and warm it. Drip it into the ear lukewarm.
3. For toothache, give the berries of this plant to eat.
4. For a bloody nose, take the juice of this same plant, dip a linen cloth
    in it, and stop up the the nostrils with it. The blood will soon stop.

77. Common Groundsel (*Senecio vulgaris L.*), *senecio*, *Grundeswylge*

This plant, which is called *senecio* or groundsel, grows on roofs and along
walls.

1. For wounds, even if they are fairly old, take the plant that we call
    senecio [groundsel], pound it with aged lard, lay it on the wounds,
    and they will heal quickly.
2. If anyone has been struck with iron, pick the same plant in early
    morning or the middle of the day, pound it, as we said earlier, with
    aged lard, lay it on the cut, and quickly it opens and purges the
    wound.
3. For gout, take the same plant, pound it with lard, put it on the foot,
    and it will relieve the pain. Also, this helps a great deal for painful
    joints.

---

196. C, DeV = *Atropa belladona*, and D'A accepts this reading as well. Both belong to the
Solanacal family.
197. C says this is oil of privet, and that cyprus was the medical name for privet.

4. For sore loins, take this same plant, pound it with salt just as you would for a poultice, and put it on the loins. The same thing helps for sore feet.

78. Fern (*Felix L.*), *felix, Fearn*

1. For wounds, take the pounded roots of the plant we call *felix* or fern and lay them on the wound. Also give about nine grams of stitchwort to drink in wine.
2. If a young man is ruptured, take the same plant (one growing in the roots of a beech tree), pound it with lard, spread a cloth with it, and fasten this to the sore so that the cloth is always turned upward. On the fifth day he will be well.

79. Couch Grass (*Cynodon dactylon*), *gramen, Cwice*[198]

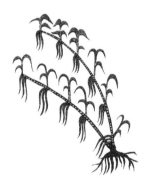

1. For pain in the spleen, take the leaves of the plant that is called *gramen* or couch grass, and simmer them. Apply this to a cloth and lay it on the spleen. You will perceive benefit from this.

80. Iris (*Iris L.*), *gladiolus, Glædene*[199]

1. For pain in the bladder and if a person cannot urinate, take the outer part of the roots of the plant that is called *gladiolus* [iris], dry it, pound it, and mix with it two cups of wine and three cups of water. Give this to drink.

---

198. D'A accepts André's reasoning that the "grass that has three branches" mentioned in the Latin description and shown clearly in the manuscript illustration is couch grass, not quitch (*Agropyrum repens L.*) suggested by C and DeV.
199. D'A accepts André's identification without comment; C and DeV = yellow flag *(Iris pseudacorus L.)*

2. For pain of the spleen, take the same plant when it is young, dry it and pound it into powder. Give this to drink in light wine. It is believed that it will heal the spleen in a wonderful manner.

3. For abdominal and chest[200] pain, take the pounded berries of this plant and give them to drink in goat's milk or better in lukewarm wine. The soreness will go away.

81. Rosemary (*Rosmarinus officinalis L.*), rosmarinum, Boþen

This plant, called *rosmarinum* or rosemary, grows in sandy soil and in gardens.[201]

1. For toothache, take the root of the plant we call *rosmarinum* [rosemary] and give it to eat. Without delay, it will relieve the toothache. If the juice is held in the mouth, it will quickly heal the teeth.

2. For the sickly, take the plant *rosmarinum* [rosemary], pound it with oil, and rub it on the person. You will heal him wonderfully.

3. For itching, take the same plant, pound it, and mix its juice with aged wine and warm water. Give it to drink for three days.

4. For liver and abdominal disease, take a handful of this same plant, pound it into water, and mix with it two handfuls of spikenard and some stalks of rue. Simmer together in water and give to drink. The person will get better.

5. For fresh wounds, take the same plant we call *rosmarinum* [rosemary], pound it with lard, and lay it onto the wound.

82. Wild Carrot or Parsnip (*Daucus carota L.* or *Pastinaca sativa L*), pastinaca siluatica, Feldmoru

This plant, which is called *pastinace siluatice* or wild carrot, grows in sandy soils and on hills.

1. If a woman has difficulty in giving birth, take the plant we call *pastinaca siluatica* [wild carrot or parsnip], simmer it in water, and give it so that she can bathe herself with it. She will be healed.

2. For a woman's cleansing, take the same plant, *pastinaca* [wild carrot or parsnip], simmer it in water, and when it is soft, mix it well and give it to drink. She will be cleansed.

---

200. *breost*, which can be chest or breasts. C = breasts. The Latin (*praecordia*) would favor chest.
201. The Old English term, *wyrtbett*—plant bed or garden plot—supports the idea that many of these plants were grown in special beds, as discussed in chapter 3.

83. Pellitory-of-the-Wall (*Parietaria officinalis L.*), *perdicalis, Dolhrune*

This plant, called *perdicalis* or pellitory-of-the-wall, grows along roads, against walls, and on hills.

1. For gout and ulcerous sores, take this plant that we call *perdicalis* [pellitory-of-the-wall] and simmer it in water. Bathe the feet and the knees with it. Then pound the plant with lard, make it into a poultice, and lay it onto the feet and the knees. You will heal the person.

84. Mercury (*Mercurialis perennis L.*), *mercurialis, Cedelc*

1. For constipation, take this plant that one calls *mercurialis* or mercury, crumbled in water. Give this to the sufferer and quickly the constipation will be driven out, and the stomach will be purged. The seed cures in the same manner.
2. For pain and swelling of the eyes, take the pounded leaves of this same plant in old wine and lay them on the swollen eyes.
3. If water gets into the ears, take lukewarm juice of this plant and drip it into the ear. Soon the water will dissipate.

85. Polypody (*Polypodium vulgare L.*), *radiola, Eforfearn*

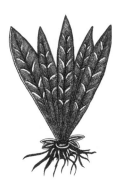

This plant, which is called *radiolus* or polypody, is like a fern, and it grows in stony places and on ruins. It has on each leaf two rows of beautiful spots, and they shine like gold.

1. For headache, take the plant that we call *radiolus* [polypody] and clean it very well. Simmer it in vinegar and smear the head with it. It will relieve the headache.

86. Asparagus (*Asparagus officinalis L.*), *herba sparagiagrestis,*
Wuduceruille[202]

   1. For pain or swelling of the bladder, take the roots of the plant that is
      called *sparagiagrestis* or asparagus, simmer it down in water by
      three-fourths, then drink it for seven days on an empty stomach.
      Baths should be taken for many days—the patient is not to get in or
      drink cold water—and he will feel healthy in a wonderful way.
   2. For toothache, take the juice of this same plant, which we call
      sparagi [asparagus], give it to drink and to hold (some of it) in the
      mouth.
   3. For sore veins, take the roots of this same plant pounded with wine
      and give them to drink. It helps.
   4. If any ill-meaning person enchants another out of spite, take the
      dried roots of this same plant, give them to eat with well water, and
      sprinkle the person with the water. The person will be freed from the
      enchantment.

87. Savine (*Juniperus sabina L.*), *sabine, Sauine*

   1. For the king's evil,[203] which is called *aurignem* in Latin and means
      painful joints and foot swelling in our language, take this plant,
      which is called savine, and by other names similar to savine, give it
      to drink with honey. It will relieve the pain. It does the same thing
      mixed with wine.
   2. For headache, take the same plant, savine, well pounded in vinegar
      and mixed with oil. Rub it on the head and the temples. It will help
      remarkably.
   3. For carbuncles, take the savine plant mixed with honey and smear it
      on the sore.

88. Small Snapdragon (*Antirrhinum orontium L.*), *canis caput, Hundes
Heafod*

   1. For soreness and swelling of the eyes, take the roots of this plant,
      which is called *canis caput* in Latin and in our language snapdragon,
      simmer them in water, and then bathe the eyes with the water. It will
      quickly soothe the pain.

---

202. DeV and Bierbaumer = wild chervil (*Anthriscus silvestris*); D'A says chervil has no medicinal properties, and accepts André's suggestion that this is asparagus, which has many medicinal properties, especially as a diuretic.
203. *wiþ þa cynelican adle.* Literally, "king's evil"which DeV and the DOE note was a condition
that the king could cure, here, jaundice, particularly jaundice associated with gout. C uses the
Latin, *ad morbum regium,* in his translation. See Marc Bloch, *The Royal Touch: Sacred Monarchy and Scrofula in England and France,* trans. J. E. Anderson (London: Routledge & Kegan
Paul, 1973).

89. Blackberry or Bramble (*Rubus fruticosus L.*), *erusti, Bremel*

1. For earache, take the plant that is called *erusti* or blackberry when soft and pound it. Then take the juice, lukewarm, and drip it into the ear. It lessens the pain and effectively heals.
2. For a woman's menstrual flow, take the berries of this same plant when they are soft—take three times seven of them[204]—and simmer them down in water by two-thirds. Give this to drink on an empty stomach for three days; but make a new drink each day.
3. For heart pain, take the leaves of this plant pounded by themselves. Lay them on the left nipple. The pain will go away.
4. For fresh wounds, take the flowers of this same plant and lay them on the wounds. It will heal the wounds without any delay or danger.
5. For a pain in the joints, take some of this same plant and simmer it down in wine by two-thirds. Bathe the joints with this wine, and all the disease in the joints will be relieved.
6. For snakebite, take the leaves of the same plant that we call *erusti*, freshly pounded, and lay them on the bite.

90. Yarrow (*Achillea millefolium L.*), *millefolium, Gearwe*

1. About the plant that is called *millefolium* and in our language yarrow, it is said that Lord Achilles discovered it, and that with this same plant he cured those who were cut by an iron weapon and were wounded. It is also said some men named it *achillea* because of this, and also that it cured a man named Thelephos.
2. For toothache, take the roots of this same plant that we call *millefolium* [yarrow]. Give them to eat on an empty stomach.
3. For wounds that have been caused by something made of iron, take the same plant pounded in lard and smear it on the wounds. It will cleanse and heal the wounds.
4. For swellings, take the same plant, *millefolium* [yarrow], pounded in butter. Smear it on the swelling.
5. If someone has difficulty urinating, take the juice of this same plant with vinegar and give it to drink. It cures wonderfully.
6. If a wound has cooled, take the same plant, *millefolium* [yarrow], pound it small, and mix it with butter. Put this on the wound; it will quickly recover feeling and warm up.
7. If someone's head breaks out in rashes, or strange swellings appear on the face, take the roots of this same plant and fasten them around the neck. This will benefit him greatly.

---

204. In case any numerology is involved in the directions, the instructions are translated as given. The Latin reads *ter septenas.*

8. For the same condition, take the same plant, powder it, put it on the sores, and soon they will become slightly inflamed.[205]

9. If the veins have hardened or digestion is difficult, take the juice of this same plant; mix wine, water, and honey together with the juice. Give this to the patient to drink warm and he will quickly improve.

10. Again for intestinal and abdominal pain, take the same plant and dry it, then make it into a fine powder. Put five spoonfuls of the powder into three cups[206] of good wine. Give this to the person to drink. This will benefit any internal condition.

11. If the person develops hiccoughs or heartburn after taking that, take the roots of this same plant and pound them well. Put them in good beer and give this to drink lukewarm. I expect that it will truly benefit, both for hiccoughs or for any other painful internal condition.

12. For headache, take the same plant, make a poultice with it, and smear it on the head. It will quickly take the pain away.

13. For bites of the kind of snake called "splangius," take twigs and leaves of the same plant, simmer them in wine, pound them up fine, and apply this to the bite to help close it up. Then take the plant and honey, mix them together, apply this to the bite, and it will quickly become slightly inflamed and heal.

14. To prevent snake and spider bites: If anyone wears this plant and carries it with him on his way, he will be shielded from every kind of snake and spider.

15. For bite of a mad dog, take the same plant and grind it and wheat seeds. Put them on the bite, and this will quickly heal it.

16. Again, for snakebite, if the wound is swollen, take twigs of this same plant, simmer them in water, grind them very small, and lay them soaking wet on the wound. When the cut is open, take the same plant, dry, pound it very small, mix it with honey, and treat the wound with it. It will quickly heal.

91. Rue (*Ruta graveolens L.*), rute, Rude

1. For nosebleed, take the plant that is called *ruta* or rue and put it in the nostrils often. It controls the nosebleed in a wonderful manner.

2. For swellings, take the same plant, *ruta* [rue], give it fresh a little at a time to eat or in a drink.

3. For stomachache, take the seeds of this same plant, sulphur, and vinegar. Give this to eat on an empty stomach.

---

205. Slight inflammation is a sign a sore is beginning to heal.
206. The Old English does not have cups here, just "three of wine," but this is a customary proportion of plant to liquid. Six spoonfuls of dried plant and three spoonfuls of liquid would not be usual. The Latin original is not given.

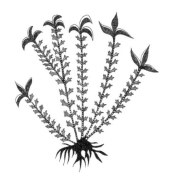

4. For eye pain and swelling, take the same plant, *ruta* [rue], pounded well, and lay it on the sore eyes. Also the pounded roots smeared on cure the pain very well.

5. For the illness that is called *lithargum*, and in our language forgetfulness, take the same plant, *ruta* [rue], soaked in vinegar. Sprinkle it on the temples.

6. For dimness of the eyes, take the leaves of this same plant, give them to eat on an empty stomach, and give them to drink in wine.

7. For headache, take the same plant and give it to drink in wine. Pound the plant and press out the juice into vinegar. Smear it on the head. The plant also helps cure carbuncles.

92. Horsemint (*Mentha longifolia* or *silvestris L.*), *mentastrus*, (*Horsminte* or *Minte*)

1. For earache, take the juice of the plant called *mentastrus* or . . . [mint] mixed with strong wine. Put this in the ear. In case worms are growing there, they should be destroyed using this.

2. For itchy skin conditions,[207] take the leaves of this same plant and give them to eat. The person will certainly be cured.

93. Dwarf Elder or Danewort (*Sambuscus ebulus L.*), *ebulus*, *Wealwyrt* or *Ellenwyrt*

1. For stones in the bladder, take the plant called *ebulus* or dwarf elder and some call danewort and pound it when its is tender. Give this to drink in wine. It will clear up the condition.

2. For snakebite, take the same plant that we call *ebulus* [dwarf elder], and before you cut it up, hold it in your hands and say this three times nine times: *Omnes malas bestias canto*, that is in our language,

---

207. DeV provides a lengthy note about the possible conditions meant by *hreofl/hreofla*, a term often used in Old English texts for various skin conditions.

enchant and overcome all evil wild beasts.[208] Cut it up into three parts with a sharp knife, and while you are doing this, think of the person you want to cure using it. When you turn to the job, do not look around and about—be focused. Take the plant and pound it, then lay it on the bite. The person will recover quickly.

3. For dropsy, take the pounded roots of this same plant, wring out enough from it so that you have four cups and add it to a half jug of wine. Give this to drink all in one day, and it will greatly help the dropsy.

Also, within half a year, it will expel all the fluids caused by the dropsy.

94. Pennyroyal (*Mentha pulegium L.*), *pollegium, Dweorgedwosle*[209]

This plant, called *pollegium* or pennyroyal, effects many cures, although many do not know them, because this plant is of two kinds, that is, masculine and feminine. The masculine variety has white flowers, and the feminine red or brown; both are beneficial, wondrous, and have wondrous powers. They bloom with the brightest color just about when other plants are withering and fading.

1. For abdominal pain, take the *pollegium* [pennyroyal] plant and caraway, pound them together with water and place this on the navel. It will quickly be cured.
2. Again, for stomachache, take the same plant, *pollegium* [pennyroyal], pound it, and rinse it with water. Give it to drink in vinegar. It will relieve the stomach pain very well.
3. For genital itching, take the same plant, simmer in gently boiling water, and then let it cool until one can drink it. Drink it, and it will relieve the itching.
4. Again, for abdominal pain: this plant relieves it well when eaten and placed on the navel so that it cannot fall off. It will quickly alleviate the pain.
5. For tertian fever, take branches of this same plant, enfold them in wool, and fumigate the patient with it before the fever is due to strike. If you fasten this plant around the head, the person's headache will be relieved.
6. If a stillborn child is inside a woman, take three sprigs of this plant, so fresh that they have a strong smell, pound them in aged wine, and give this to drink.

---

208. For many who collect plants in the wild (wildcrafters) and herbalists, speaking to a plant before it is cut explaining why one is gathering it is not at all unusual.
209. DeV has a note on the meaning of *dweorgedwosle* and the role dwarfs were thought to play in causing disease and fever.

7. For seasickness, take the same plant, *pollegium* [pennyroyal], and wormwood. Pound them together with oil and vinegar and rub the person with it often.

8. For bladder pain and for the stones that develop there, take the same plant, *pollegium* [pennyroyal], pounded well and two cups of wine. Mix them together and give this to drink. The bladder will quickly become much better, and within a few days it will cure the condition, and the stones that developed will be expelled.

9. If anyone experiences pain around the heart or chest, the person should eat of this same plant, *pollegium* [pennyroyal], and drink of it on an empty stomach.

10. If anyone suffers from a cramp, take the same plant and two cups of vinegar, and drink this on an empty stomach.

11. For swelling of the abdomen and intestinal swelling, take this same plant, *pollegium* [pennyroyal], pounded and simmered in wine or water, or give it to eat by itself. The discomfort will be relieved quickly.

12. For pain of the spleen, take the same plant, *pollegium* [pennyroyal], and simmer it in vinegar. Give it to drink warm.

13. For pain of the loins or thighs, take equal amounts of this same plant, *pollegium* [pennyroyal], and pepper and mix them together. When you are bathing, apply this where it hurts the most.

95. Nepeta (*Mentha solvestris*), nepitamon, Nepte[210]

This plant is called *nepitamon* or catmint, and the Greeks call it *menthe orinon.*

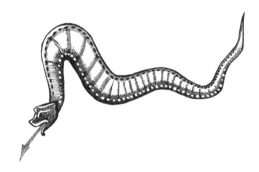

1. For snakebite, take the plant that we call *nepitamon*, pound it in wine, wring out the juice, and give it to drink in wine. Then take the pounded leaves of the same plant and lay them on the wound.

---

210. DeV = Catmint (*Nepeta cataria L.*). *Nepeta* belongs to the same family as mints, the *Labiatae*.

96. Hog's Fennel or Sulphurwort (*Peucedanum officinale L.*), *peucedana, Cammoc*

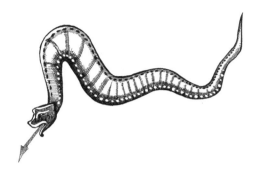

The plant is called *peucedana* or hog's fennel.

1. This plant, which we call *peucedana* [hog's fennel], can make snakes flee by its smell.
2. For snakebite, take the same plant, *peucedana* [hog's fennel], *betonica* [betony], deer's grease or marrow, and vinegar. Mix this together and smear it on the wound; it will heal.
3. For the disease the Greeks call *frenesis*, which is witlessness of the mind in our language, that is, when the head becomes very hot, take the same plant, *peucedana* [hog's fennel], pound it in vinegar, and sprinkle the head with this. It heals very well.

97. Elecampane (*Inula helenium L.*), *hinnula campana, Sperewyrt*

1. For bladder pain, take this plant called *hinnula campana* or elecampane, wild celery seed, asparagus, and fennel root, pound them together, and give this to drink lukewarm.[211] It heals with certainty.
2. For toothache and loose teeth, take the same plant and give it to eat on an empty stomach. It firms up the teeth.
3. If intestinal worms are seen around the anus, take the same plant, *hinnula* [elecampane], pound it in wine, and lay it on the abdomen.

---

211. Probably to drink in water or wine.

98. Hound's-Tongue *(cynoglossum officinale)* [Narrow-Leaved Plantain or Ribwort *(Plantago lanceolata L.)*], *cynoglossa, Ribbe*[212]

The plant is called *cynoglossa* or ribwort and sometimes hound's-tongue.

1. For snakebite, the plant that we call *cynoglossa* [hound's-tongue] cures well when pounded and taken in wine.
2. For quartan fever, take this same plant, *cynoglossa* [hound's-tongue], the one with four leaves, pound it, and give it to drink in water. It will cure the person.
3. If the ears don't work right, and if a person can't hear well, take the same plant, *cynoglossa* [hound's-tongue], pounded and warmed in oil. Drip it into the ear, and it will help in a wonderful manner.

99. Saxifrage *(Saxifraga granulata L.)*, s*axifraga, Sundcorn*

The plant called *saxifraga* or saxifrage grows on hills and in rocky places.

1. For stones in the bladder, take the plant we call *saxifraga* [saxifrage], pound it in wine, and give in warm water to anyone suffering and feverish. It is so effective, that of it is said: whoever tries it, it will break up their stones on that same day and it will expel them, and will lead to their health.

100. Ivy *(Hedera helix L.)*, *hedera nigra, Eoreifig*[213]

1. For stones in the bladder, take seven to eleven berries of the plant that is called *hedera nigra* or ivy crushed in water. Give this to drink. It will collect the stones in the bladder in a wondrous way and will destroy them and send them out through the urine.
2. For headache, take the same plant, *hedera* [ivy], and rose juice soaked in wine. Rub this on the temples and the face, and the pain will lessen.
3. For pain in the spleen, on the first attack, take three berries of this same plant, on the next, five; at the third attack take seven; at the fourth time, nine; at the fifth, eleven; at the sixth, thirteen; and the seventh time fifteen; at the eighth, seventeen; and at the ninth, nineteen; and at the tenth, twenty-one. Give to drink daily in wine, but if there is fever present, give it in warm water. Great improvement and strength will result.

---

212. The Old English name of the plant in the manuscripts corresponds to the plant pictured in the Cotton manuscript; however D'A notes that the original Latin sources for this remedy refer to hound's-tongue, not to plantain.
213. Bierbaumer and DeV = *Glechoma hederaceum*, ground-ivy.

4. For the bite of the spider called "spalangiones,"[214] take the juice of the roots of the same plant we call *hedera* [ivy] and give it to drink.
5. To treat wounds, take the same plant, simmer it in wine, and lay it on the wound.
6. If the nostrils smell bad, take the juice of this same plant, clarified, and pour it into the nostrils.
7. If the ears do not work well and if one does not hear well, take the juice of this same plant, very clean, with wine, and drip this into the ears. The person will be healed.
8. So that the head will not ache because of the sun's heat, take the soft part of the leaves of this plant, pound them in vinegar, and smear this on the face. It also prevents any other pain that bothers the head.

101. Wild Thyme (*Thymus serpillum L.*), *serpillus, Organe*

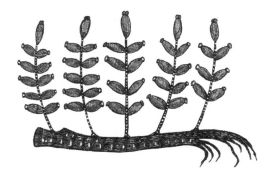

1. For headache, take the juice of the plant called *serpillus* or wild thyme, oil, and burned salt made into a fine powder. Mix everything together, smear the head with this, and it will be healed.
2. Again, for headache, take the same plant, *serpillus* [wild thyme], simmered. Pound it in vinegar and smear it on the temples and the face.
3. For bad burns, take the same plant, *serpillus* [wild thyme], one stalk of vervain, one ounce of silver shavings, and three ounces of roses. Pound all of these in a mortar, add wax to this, and half a pound of bear and deer grease. Simmer this together, purify it, and smear it on the burns.

---

214. DeV has a note about what kind of spider this may have been, pointing out that the Latin name is always used. The same Latin name is used for a snake in other places. A venomous bite from a spider or snake could have been treated in a similar manner. C = tarantula.

102. Wormwood (*Artemisia absinthium L.*), *absinthius, Wermod*

This plant, which is called *absinthium* or wormwood, grows in cultivated soil, on hills, and in rocky places.

1. For removing bruises and other sores from the body, take the plant *absinthium* [wormwood], simmer it in water, put it in a cloth, and put it on the sore. If the flesh is tender, simmer it in honey and lay it on the sore.

2. If worms are a bother around the anus, take equal amounts of the same plant, *absinthium* [wormwood], horehound, and lupine. Simmer them in sweetened water or in wine. Put it on the anus two or three times, and it will kill the worms.

103. Sage (*Salvia officinalis L.*), *salfia, Saluie*

1. For genital[215] itching, take the plant called *salvia* [sage], simmer it in water, and smear it on the genitals.

2. For itching of the anus, take the same plant, *salvia* [sage], simmer it in water, and bathe the anus with the water. It relieves the itching very well.

104. Coriander (*Coriandrum sativum L.*), *coliandra, Celendre*

1. For worms around the anus, take the plant called *coliandrum* or coriander, simmer it down in oil by two-thirds, and put it on the sores and also on the head.

2. So that a woman may give birth quickly, take eleven or thirteen seeds of this same *coliandra* [coriander] plant, bind them with a thread to a clean linen cloth, take a person who is a virgin,[216] a boy or a girl, and let them hold it at the left thigh near the genitals. As soon as the entire process of birth is completed, take the remedy away immediately, so that some of the intestines do not follow.

105. Wild Purslane (*Portulaca oleracea L.*), *porclaca*, no OE word

1. For excessive flow of semen,[217] the plant that is called *porclaca* or . . . [purslane] helps effectively, either eaten by itself or with other drinks.

---

215. *gescapa*. C = shapes (or the *verenda*). In the next entry, C calls the anus "settle," retaining the Old English word.

216. *nime ðonne an man þe sy mægðhades man, cnapa oþþe mægden*: literally, "take then a person who is a virginal person, boy or girl," illustrating at least one instance in the text of Old English *man* clearly indicating "a person" and not the modern English "a man."

217. *wiþ swiðlichne flewsan þæs sædes*. C = for violent gonorrhœa. Neither DeV or BT have a note that this is the condition meant here.

106. Chervil (*Anthriscus cerefolium L.*), *cerefolia, Cerfille*

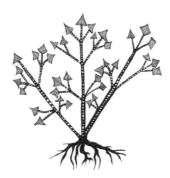

1. For stomachache, take three green sprouts from the plant called *cere-folium* or chervil, and pennyroyal. Grind them well in a wooden mor-tar together with one spoonful refined honey and fresh poppy.[218] Simmer them together and give this to eat. It will quickly strengthen the stomach.

107. Brook or Water Mint (*Mentha acquatica* or *hirsuta L.*), *sisimbrius,* *Brocminte*

1. For bladder pain and for inability to urinate, take the juice of this plant that is called *sisimbrium* or brook mint, give this to the person who is ill to drink in warm water if feverish, or if not, give it in wine. You will cure him wondrously.

108. Alexanders or Horse Parsley (*Smyrnium olusatrum L.*), *olisatrum,* no OE name

1. Again, for bladder pain and inability to urinate, take the plant we call *olisatrum* [alexanders or horse parsely], pound it into simmered wine and give it to drink. It greatly improves the ability to urinate.

109. Lily (*Lilium spp. L.*), *erinion, Lilie*

This plant is called *erinion* or lilie.

1. For snakebite, take the plant that we call lily and bulbs of the plant we call narcissus,[219] pound them together, and give this to drink. Take the pounded bulb of this plant, lay it on the bite, and it will heal.

---

218. *ameredes hiniges 7 grene popig.* C = spoilt honey and a green poppy. *Grene* is used to mean fresh many times in this work.
219. C and DeV note that the translator made a mistake here and translated the Latin *lilii bulbum* (bulb of the lily) as two different plants.

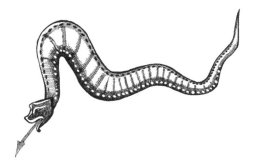

2.   For swellings, take a pounded lily leaf and lay it on the swelling. It will certainly cure it and reduce the swelling.

110. Caper-Spurge (*Euphorbia lathyris*), *titlmallos calatites*, no OE name

This plant, which is called *titymallos calatites* or caper-spurge, grows in wet places and on the shore.

1.   For abdominal pain, take a shoot of the plant *titymalli,* pound it into wine so that there are two cups of wine, add to it two spoonfuls of the juice of this plant, and give this to drink on an empty stomach. It will heal the person.
2.   For warts, take the milky sap from this plant and the juice of celery-leaved crowsfoot and put it on the warts. On the third day, it will cure the warts.
3.   For skin irritations,[220] take the flowers of this same plant simmered in resin and apply it.

111. Sow-Thistle (*Sonchus oleraceus L.*), *carduum silfaticum, Wudueistel*

This plant, called *carduum silfaticum* or sow-thistle, grows in meadows and along roadways.

1.   For stomachache, take the upper part of the flower-head of the plant we call *carduum silfaticum* [sow-thistle] when it is soft and fresh, and give this to eat in sweetened vinegar. It will cure the soreness.
2.   So that you will not fear that any evil will come near you,[221] pick this same plant, *carduum silfaticum* [sow-thistle], at daybreak when the sun first comes up—let it be when the moon is in Capricorn— and keep it with you. As long as you bear it on you, no evil will come to you.

---

220. *hreofl.* C = leprosy. The term applies to a wide variety of skin rashes and irritations.
221. *wiþ þæt ðu nane yfele gean cymas ðe ne ondræde.* C = In order that thou may dread no ill gaincomers.

112. Lupin (*Lupinus L.*), *lupinus montanus*, no OE word[222]

This plant, which is called *lupinus montanus* or . . . [lupin], grows along hedges and in sandy places.

1.   For intestinal worms that irritate around the anus take the *lupinus montanus* [lupine] plant, pounded, and give it to drink in one cup of vinegar. Without delay it will drive out the worms.
2.   If the same thing bothers children, take the same plant, lupine, and wormwood, pound them together and put this on the anus.

113. Spurge laurel or spurge flax (*Daphne laureola L.* or *D. Gnidium L.*), *lactyrida, Givcorn*

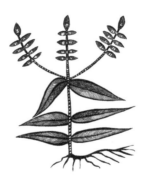

This plant, which is called *lactyrida* or spurge laurel, grows in cultivated and sandy soils.

1.   For constipation, take the seeds of this plant (they are the berries) well washed. Give this to drink in warm water. It will soon move the intestines.

114. Lettuce (*Chondrilla juncea L.*), *lactuca leporina,* no OE word[223]

This plant, which is called *lactuca* [lettuce], grows in cultivated and in sandy soils. About this plant, it is said that the hare, when it is tired in the summer from the heat, heals itself with this same plant. Because of this, it is named "hare's lettuce" in Latin.

---

222. C, DeV, Bierbaumer = *Lupinus albus.*
223. Bierbaumer, DeV = *Lactuca virosa L.*

1. For feverishness, take the *lactuca leporina* [lettuce] plant and lay it under a person's pillow without his knowing it. The person will be cured.

115. Squirting cucumber (*Ecballium elaterium Rich.*), cucumeris siluatica, Hwerhwette[224]

This plant, called *cucumeris siluatica* or cucumber, grows near the sea and in hot places.

1. For sore joints and for gout, take the root of this plant that we call *cucumeris silfatica* [cucumber], simmer it down in oil by two-thirds, and smear it on.
2. If a child is born prematurely or misshapen, take the roots of this same plant simmered down by two thirds and wash the child with it. Also, if anyone eats the fruit of this plant on an empty stomach, he will be endangered; for that reason, everyone should restrain from eating it on an empty stomach.[225]

116. Hemp (*Cannabis sativa L.*), cannaue silfatica, Henep

This plant, which is called *cannane silfatica* or hemp, grows in rough places, along roads and hedges.

1. For sore breasts, take the hemp plant pounded in lard, lay it on the breasts, and it will diminish the swelling. If any inflammation is present, it will clear it up.
2. For frostbite, take the fruit of this same plant pounded with nettle seeds and soaked in vinegar, and put it on the sore.

117. Wild Rue (*Ruta montana*), ruta montana, Rude

This plant, called *ruta montana* or rue, grows on hills and uncultivated places.

1. For dim eyesight and for bad scars, take the leaves of the plant we call *ruta montana* [rue] simmered in aged wine. Put this in a glass vessel, and then smear it on.
2. For a sore chest,[226] take the same plant, *ruta siluatica* [rue], and pound it in a wooden vessel. Then take as much as you can pick up with three fingers, put it into a pot, and add to it one cup of wine and

---

224. According to D'A, this cucumber is a wild species that grows near the sea in warm places. Bierbaumer, DeV = cucumber (*cucumis sativus L.*).

225. The directions here appear to be an indirectly stated method to terminate the life of a premature or misformed newborn.

226. Although the Latin differentiates between women's breasts (*mamilla*) and the chest/breast as seat of the heart (*praecordia*), the Old English does not. The remedy seems to be more for chest pain than for sore breasts (take the drink and rest). In either case, the drink is supposed to soothe the person. *Wiþ ðære breostan sare.* C = sore of the breasts.

two of water. Give this to drink and let the person rest for awhile; the person will be better quickly.

3. For liver pain, take a handful of this plant, a jug and a half of water, and the same amount of honey. Simmer this together and give it to drink for three days, more if the person needs it. You will have the power to cure him.

4. If one cannot urinate, take nine stalks of this same *ruta siluatica* [rue] and three cups of water; pound [the rue] and mix, then add half a jug of vinegar. Simmer them together and then give this to drink continually for nine days. The person will be cured.

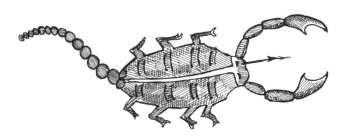

5. For bites of the snake that is called a scorpion, take the seeds of the plant called *ruta siluatica* [rue], pound them in wine, and give it to drink. It will alleviate the pain.

118. Tormentil (*Potentilla theptaphylla L.* or *Potentilla recta L.*), *septifolium, Seofenleafe*

This plant, which is called *eptafilon* or *septifolium* or tormentil, grows in gardens and in sandy soil.

1. For gout, take the *septifolium* [tormentil] plant pounded and mixed with saffron. Smear the juice on the feet. In three days the pain will be taken away.

119. Basil or Wild Basil (*Ocimum basilicum* or *Calaminthe vulgare L.*), *ocimus, Mistel*

1. For headache, take the plant called *ocimum* or basil, pound it with rose or myrtle juice or with vinegar and lay it on the face.

2. For eye pain and swelling, pound this same plant into good wine and smear this on the eyes. You will heal them.

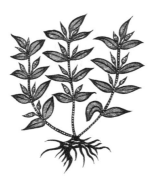

3.   For kidney pain, do the same thing and give it to drink with the skin of apples that are named *mala granata*.[227]

120. Wild Celery (*Apium graveolens L.*), *apium, Merce*

1.   For eye pain and swelling, take the plant called *apium* or wild celery pounded well with bread and lay it on the eyes.

121. Ivy (*Hedera chrysocaspa Walsh*), *hedera, Ifig*

This plant, which is called *crysocantes* or ivy, is called *crysocantes* because it bears seeds that are like gold.

1.   For dropsy, take twenty seeds of this plant, crush them into a jug of wine. Give three cups of this wine to drink for seven days; the disease will be expelled through the urine.

122. Mint (*Mentha spp. L.*), *menta, Minte*[228]

1.   For impetigo and pimples, take the juice of the plant called *mentha* or mint; add to it sulphur and vinegar, and pound everything together. Apply it with a feather, and the sores will improve quickly.
2.   If bad scars or cuts are on the head, take the same plant, mint, pounded. Lay it on the sores, and it will heal them.

123. Dill (*Anethum graveolens L.*), *annetum, Dile*

1.   For genital itching or soreness, take the plant that is called *anetum* or dill, burn it into dust, then take the dust and honey and mix it together. First bathe the sore place with warm myrtle-tree water, and then apply the preparation.

---

227. C says this is a pomegranate. Mālum is apple in Latin.
228. Bierbaumer = field mint *(mentha arvensis L.).*

2. If the same thing troubles a woman, her midwife should provide the same remedy for her as we said earlier.
3. For headache, take the flowers of the same plant and simmer them with oil. Apply this to the temples and fasten it to the head.

124. Wild Marjoram or Sweet Marjoram (*Origanum vulgare* or *majorana L.*), *origanum, Organe*

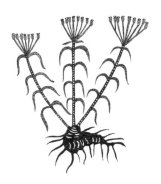

1. This plant, called *origanum* or marjoram, has a hot, violent nature and it breaks up coughs and bad blood. It subdues gout and cures shortness of breath and liver sickness very well.
2. For coughs, take the same plant, marjoram, and give it to eat. You will be surprised at its effects.

125. Houseleek *(Sempervivum arboreum L.), semperuiuus, Sinfulle*

1. For accumulations of fluids in the body, take the plant that is called *sempervivum* or houseleek, lard, bread, and coriander. Pound them together as you would make a poultice and lay this on the infected place.

126. Fennel *(Foeniculum vulgare), fenuculus, Finul*

1. For coughing and shortness of breath, take the roots of the plant called *fenuculus* or fennel, pound it in wine, and drink it on an empty stomach for nine days.
2. For bladder pain, take a handful of the same plant, which we call fennel, when fresh, and fresh roots of wild celery and of asparagus, and put them in a new earthenware pot with one jug of water. Simmer down by three fourths. Let the person drink this on an empty stomach for seven days or more, and let him take a bath, however not a

cold one, nor should cold water be drunk. The bladder pain will be relieved without delay.

127. Rue *(Ruta chalepensis L.), erifion, Liðwort*[229]

This plant, *erifion* or rue, was originally grown in Gaul, that is France, on the mountain called Soractis. It looks like wild celery, has red flowers like garden cress, and it has seven roots and the same number of stems. It propagates itself in uncultivated places, but not moist ones. It blooms at all times and has seeds like beans.

1. For lung disease, take the rue plant, pounded as for making a poultice. Lay this on the sore spot, and it will heal it. Then take the juice of this same plant, give it to drink, and you will be surprised at the power of this plant.

128. Comfrey *(Symphytum officinale* or *orientale* or *tauricum L.), sinfitus albus, Halswyrt*[230]

1. For a woman's menses, take the plant called *sinfitus albus* or comfrey, dry it, and pound it into fine powder. Give it to drink in wine, and the flow will quickly cease.

129. Parsley *(Petroselinum hortense Huff.), petrosilinum, Petersilie*

The plant is called *triannem* or *petroselinum,* and some call it parsley.

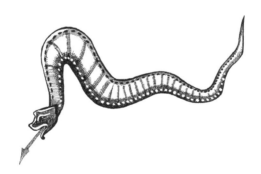

1. For snakebite, take four grams of the *petroselini* plant [parsley] made into very fine powder and give this to drink in wine. Then take the pounded plant and lay it on the wound.

---

229. DeV gives goat's rue, *Galega officinalis,* for this plant.
230. De V gives common ash, *Fraximus excelsior L.* C originally proposed that it was a *Symphytum.* Bierbaumer does not positively identify this plant.

2. For nerve pain, take the same plant, parsley, pounded, lay it on the painful place, and it will quickly heal the nerve pain.

130. Cabbage or Colewort (Brassica oleracea L. or napus L.), brassica, Caul or Cawel

1. For any swelling, take the shoots of the plant called *brassica siluatica* or cabbage, pound and mix them with aged lard, and make this as you would a poultice. Put this onto a thick linen cloth and lay it on the sore.
2. For a pain in the side, take the same *brassica siluatica* plant [cabbage], and put it on the sore mixed as we just told you.
3. For gout, take the same *brassica siluatica* plant [cabbage], mixed the same way we said earlier. The longer the preparation stands, the more effective and healing it will be.

131. Sweet Basil (Ocimum basilicum L.), basilisca, Nædderwyrt

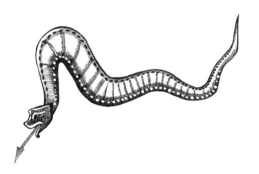

1. This plant, called *basilisca* or basil, grows where the snake is that has the same name, *basiliscus*.[231] Indeed, there is not one kind of basil, but three. One is olocryseis, that is, as said in our language, that it shines like gold. Another kind is *stillatus*, which is "spotted" in our language; it looks as though its head were golden. The third kind is *sanguineus*, that is blood-red, and also looks as if its head were golden. The basil plant comes in all these kinds. If anyone has this plant with him, none of the following kinds of snakes can harm him. The *olocryssuss* snake is named *eriseos*, and whatever it sees it blows on and sets on fire. The second, *stillatus*, is called *crysocefalus aster-*

---

231. The Old English name for the plant is literally "snake plant."

ites; whatever it sees dries up and disappears. The third kind is named *hematites* or *crysocefalus*. Whatever it sees or touches it destroys so that nothing is left but the bones. The basil plant has all of their strength, and if any person has the plant with him, that person will be strong against all kinds of snakes.

This plant is like rue: it has red milky juice like greater celandine, and it has purple flowers. Anyone who wants to pick it should purify himself and mark around it with gold and silver, with deer horn and ivory, with bear's tooth and bull's horn, and lay around it fruit sweetened with honey.

132. Mandrake *(Mandragora officinarum* or *autminalis), mandragora,* no OE word

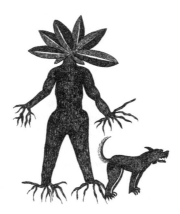

This plant called mandrake is large and glorious to see, and it is beneficial. You must gather it in this manner: when you approach the plant, and you will recognize it because it shines at night like a lantern, when you first see its head, mark around it quickly with an iron tool lest it flee from you. Its power is so great and powerful that it wants to flee quickly when an impure person approaches it.[232] Because of this, you must mark around it with an iron tool, and then you must dig around it, being careful not to touch it with the iron; however you can dig the earth strenuously with an ivory staff. When you see its hands and feet, fasten them. Take the other end and fasten it around a dog's neck (make sure the dog is hungry). Throw some meat in front of him so that he cannot reach it unless he snatches the plant up with him. About this plant it is said that it has such great powers, whatever pulls it up will quickly be deceived in the same

232. It is important to remember when reading these instructions that the root of the mandrake plant is shaped like a human being.

way. Because of this, as soon as you see that it has been pulled up, and you have power over it, immediately seize it, twist it, and wring the juice from its leaves into a glass bottle. If you need to help people with it, then help them as follows:

1. For headache and for sleeplessness, take the juice and smear it on the face, and use the plant in the same way to relieve headache. You will be surprised at how quickly sleep will come.
2. For earache, take the juice of the same plant mixed with oil of spikenard and put it into the ears. You will be surprised at how quickly it cures.
3. For gout, even if it is severe, take three pennies' weight from either the right and left hand or from either hand of this plant and powder it. Give it to drink in wine for seven days, and the person will be cured; not just that the swelling will go down, but it will also relieve nerve spasms[233] and cure pain, both in a wonderful manner.
4. For insanity, that is for possession by devils, take three pennies' weight from the body of the mandrake plant and give it to drink as easily as the person is able in warm water. He will be quickly cured.
5. Again, for nerve spasms, take one ounce by weight from the body of this plant and pound it into powder. Mix it with oil and then smear it on whomever has the aforementioned condition.
6. If anyone perceives any grievous evil in the home, take the mandrake plant to the center of the house—as much as one has of it—and it will expel all the evil.

133. Campion *(Agrostemma coronaria), lichanis stephanice, Lœcewyrt*[234]

1. This plant, which is called *lichanis stefanice* or campion, has long, luxuriant, purple leaves, its stem has luxuriant shoots, and it has yellow flowers on the upper part of the stem. The seeds of this plant given in wine help greatly against all kinds of snakes and scorpion

---

233. *þæra sina togunge.* C = the tugging of the sinews.
234. The original *Herbarium of Pseudo-Apuleius* ends at mandrake. The rest of the work is drawn from two tracts that the early-medieval world attributed to Dioscorides: *De herbis feminis* and *Curae herbarum.* See DeV, lv_lx; D'Aronco and Cameron, Introduction; and Hofstetter for a discussion of sources. Also, see J. M. Riddle, "Pseudo-Dioscorides' *Ex herbis feminis* and Early Medieval Medical Botany," *Journal of the History of Biology* 14 (1981): 43–81 for the history of this work and its long association with the Herbarium.

stings. Some say about its strength, that if a person lays it on a scorpion, it will bring the scorpion powerlessness and disease.

134. Burdock *(Arctium lappa L.), action,* no OE word

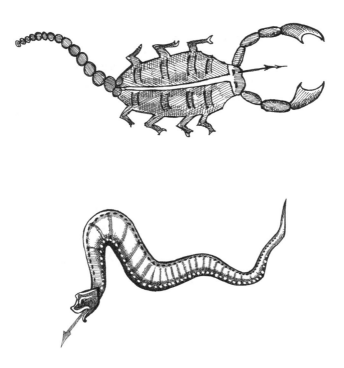

This plant, which is called *action* or burdock, has leaves like a gourd, but larger and firmer, and it has at its roots a large stalk that is more than two yards long. It has a seed like a thistle on the upper part of the stem, but it is smaller and red in color.

1. If a person coughs up blood and phlegm together, take four pennies' weight of the seeds of this plant and nuts from the cones of pine trees, and pound them together just as you make an apple dumpling. Give this to the patient, and it will cure him.
2. For pain in the joints, take the same plant, pounded and made into a poultice. Smear it on the soreness, and it will improve. It also cures old cuts in the same manner.

135. Southernwood *(Artemisia abrotanum L.), abrotanus, Sueernewuda*

There are two kinds of this plant, which is called *abrotanus* or southernwood. This one kind has large branches and very small leaves, as though they were really hairs. It has very small flowers and seeds, has a good smell, and is strong and bitter to the taste.

1. For shortness of breath, sciatica, and difficulty urinating, the seeds of this plant help if pounded and drunk in water.
2. For pain in the side, take the same plant and *betonica* [betony], pound them together, and give them to drink.
3. For poison and for snakebite, take the same plant, *abrotanus*, and give it to drink in wine. It helps very much. Also, pound it into oil and smear it on the body. It also helps cure fever chills. Moreover, the seed of this plant, scattered about or set on fire, effectively puts snakes to flight.[235]

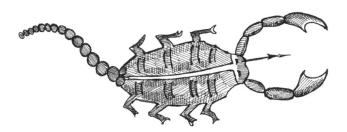

4. For a bite from snakes we call *spalangiones* or scorpion, this plant is effective.
5. For eye pain, take the same plant, *abrotanum*, simmered with the plant called *melacidonia* or quince, and mixed with bread as you would make a poultice. Apply this to the sore eyes, and the pain will be cured.

This plant is, as we said before, of two kinds: one female and one male. All have the same effects on the conditions we just listed.

136. Water Parsnip *(Sium latifolium L.), sion, Laber*

This plant, which is called *sion* or water parsnip, grows in watery places.

---

235. The Old English does not tell us what is put to flight! C supplied the word snake, which is in the Latin version.

1. For bladder stones, take the plant and give it to eat simmered or raw. It will expel the stones through the urine.
2. This plant is also effective against diarrhea and discomfort of the bowels.

137. White Heliotrope *(Heliotropium europaeum L.* or *H. Supinum L.), eliotropus, Sigilhweorfa*[236]

This plant, called *eliotropus* or heliotrope, grows in rich, cultivated soil,[237] has rough, broad leaves that are very much like wild basil, round seeds, and it comes in three colors.

1. For all kinds of snake and scorpion bites, take the roots of the *eliotropos* [heliotrope] plant, give this to drink in wine, and put it pounded on the wound. It will help a great deal.
2. For worms in the intestines [that present] around the anus, take this same plant, hyssop, salt, and watercress, and pound them together. Give this to drink in water, and it will kill the worms.
3. For warts, take the same plant and salt and pound them together. Put this on the warts, and it will take them away. For this reason, it is also called *uerrucaria* [wart plant].

138. Field Marigold *(Calendula arvensis L.), spreritis,* no OE name[238]

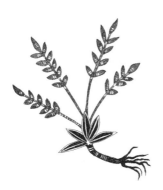

This plant, which is called *spreritis* or . . . [field marigold], has small, luxuriant leaves, and its root sends out many branches that are laid near to the ground. It has yellow flowers, and if you crush it between your fingers, it has a smell like myrrh.

---

236. All the sources consulted say it is impossible distinguish the herb described here from the one in chapter 64. C, DeV, Bierbaumer = marigold.

237. *on fættum landum 7 on beganum.* C = on fat lands and on cultivated ones.

238. C and DeV give scarlet pimpernel *(Anagallis arvensis).*

1. For fever chills, take the *speritis* plant [field marigold] and simmer it in oil. At the time the fever begins its onset, smear it on the person.
2. For the bite of a mad dog, take the same plant, pound it into a powder, then take a spoonful and give it to drink in warm water, and the person will recover.
3. For pain of the spleen, take a good handful of this same plant and a jug of milk. Simmer them together and give to drink half in the morning and half in the evening as long as the person needs it. The spleen will be healed.

139. Stonecrop *(Sedum album* or *acre L.), ayzos minor,* no OE word

This plant, which is called *ayzos minor* or . . . [stonecrop], grows along roadways and in rocky places, on hills and on old ruins. From one root, it sends out many small shoots, and it is full of many small, long, pointed, sharp, succulent leaves full of juice. Its roots are not used.

1. For impetigo, eye pain, or gout, take this plant without the roots, and pound it with fine flour in the way you would make a poultice. Apply this to the infirmity and it will cure it.
2. For headache, take the juice of this same plant and juice of roses. Mix them together and smear this on the head. The pain will lessen.
3. For bite of a *spalangione* spider, take the same *aizos* [stonecrop] plant pounded in wine and give it to drink. It heals effectively.
4. For diarrhea and intestinal discomfort and for worms that harm the intestines, this same plant will help very much.
5. For any condition of the eyes, take the juice of this same plant and smear it on the eyes. It effectively cures the condition.

140. White Hellebore *(Veratrum album L.), elleborus albus, Tunsingwyrt* or *Wedeberge*

This plant, which is called *elleborus albus* or white hellebore,[239] grows on hills, and it has leaves like a leek. The roots and the entire plant should be picked about midsummer because it is well suited to medications. To be recognized about this plant is that it has a small root, which is not so straight that it is not bent a little; it is brittle and fragile when it is dried, and when it is broken, it smells as though it sent out smoke, and it is slightly bitter to the taste. The larger roots are long, hard and very bitter to the taste, and they have the violent and dangerous power that they often choke a person quickly. As we said before, one should dry this root and cut it into lengths like peas. Ten

---

239. The translator lists two Old English names for this plant, which appears to have been highly valued in healing.

pennies' weight of this root will make many remedies for many conditions; however, it should never be given to take by itself because of its strength, but mixed with some other food in the amount commensurate with the illness, that is, if the condition is very serious, give it to drink in beer or dark, thick soup.[240]

1. For diarrhea, give this to eat in pea broth or with the plant called *oriza*[241] with flour; however, all these should be first simmered in light beer and softened.
2. Indeed, this plant cures all old, grievous, and incurable conditions, so that, even though the person thought his health was to be despaired of, he will be cured.

141. Oxeye Daisy or Marguerite *(Crysanthemum segetum), buoptalmon,* no OE word[242]

1. This plant, which is called *buoptalmon* or . . . [daisy], has tender stems and leaves like fennel, and it has yellow flowers that look like eyes, from which it got its name. It grew originally in the city of Meonia. The pounded leaves of this plant made into a poultice heal up any bad boils and callouses.
2. For damage to the body coming from an overabundance of bile, take the juice of this plant and give it to drink. It will restore the natural color, and the person will look as though coming from a hot bath.

142. Land caltrop *(Tribulus terrestris L.), tribulus, Gorst*[243]

This plant, which is called *tribulus* or land caltrop, has two varieties: one grows in gardens and the other out in the fields.

1. If the body is very hot, take this plant, pounded, and smear it on the body.
2. For swelling and putrefaction in the mouth and throat, take the *tribulus* [land caltrop] plant simmered and mixed with honey. It will heal the mouth and throat.
3. For bladder stones, take the pounded, fresh seeds of the same plant and give them to drink. It helps effectively.

---

240. *on blackan briwe.* C = black brewis. BT = a thick pottage made of meal. DeV = pottage.
241. *oriza.* C = rice. This word is not in BT or DeV.
242. DeV and D'A list several other possibilities for this plant, all of them in the *Crysanthemum* family.
243. C, DeV = gorse *(Ulex europaeus L.).* Grieve says it was not much used medicinally; however, she quotes C's description of its use against fleas (without attribution) and cites several uses for the plant, much like those given in the *Herbarium.*

4.   For snakebite, take five pennies' weight of the pounded, fresh seeds of this plant and give them to drink. In addition, take the plant with its seeds and pound it and lay it on the sore. It will drive out the poison.
5.   The seeds of this plant taken in wine help against a poisonous drink.
6.   For fleas, take the same plant simmered with its seeds and sprinkle it about the house. It kills the fleas.

143. Fleabane or Spikenard *(Conyza squarrosa* or *Inula pulicaria L.),*
conize, no OE word

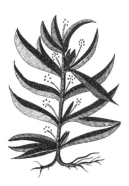

1.   This plant, which is called *conize*, has two varieties: one is large, the other small. The smaller one has small, slight leaves that smell good. The other has large, succulent leaves with an unpleasant smell, and its roots are not used. However the stem of this plant, including the leaves, if set on fire and scattered about chases away snakes. Also, when it is pounded and made into a poultice, it heals up snakebites. It also kills gnats, mosquitoes, and fleas, and cures all their bites. It stirs the urine if there is difficulty in urinating, and it cures jaundice, and helps epilepsy when given in vinegar.
2.   This plant, *conize*, simmered in water and laid under a seated woman, purifies the womb.[244]
3.   If a woman has difficulty giving birth, take the juice of this same plant soaked in wool, and put it in the genitals; it will quickly induce birth.[245]

---

244. C translates what the plant is used for into Latin.
245. This may have been originally directions for inducing an abortion, and in fact, the Latin reads that way. See Riddle, *Contraception and Abortion,* for a discussion of this topic. Because abortion was against Church teachings, Riddle says the wording for abortions was sometimes not made clear by the monks who copied and translated the texts, but the intent can be inferred. C gives the entire entry in Latin, and translates the Old English *cennan* as *parere,* to give birth. The Latin original has *abortionem praegnantibus facit.*

4. For fever chills, take the same plant and simmer in oil. Take the oil and smear it on the body. The fever will disappear.
5. For headache, take the smaller of the plants and make it into a poultice. Lay this on the soreness, and it will be relieved.

144. Thorn-Apple *(Datura stramonium L.), trycnos manicos, Foxes Glofa*[246]

1. For impetigo, take the leaf of the plant called *trycnos manicos* or thorn-apple and make it into a poultice. Smear it on the sores, and they will heal.
2. For a pimply body, which the Greeks call *erpina*, take the same plant, which we call *trycnos manicos*, and fine flour, and make it into a poultice. Apply this to the sores, and they will heal.
3. For headache, for inflammation of the stomach, and for hard swellings, take the same plant pounded in wine and smear it on the sore place. It will be healed.
4. For earache, take the juice of the same plant with juice of roses and drip it into the ear.

145. Liquorice *(Glycyrrhiza glabra L.), glycyrida,* no OE word

1. For a dry fever, take the plant called *glycyrida* or . . . [liquorice] and boil it gently in warm water. Give it to drink, and it helps effectively.
2. This plant also heals pain in the chest, liver, bladder, and kidneys when cooked and taken in wine. It also relieves thirst.
3. For diseases of the mouth, the roots of this plant eaten or drunk help the conditions.[247] It also clears up wounds that are washed with it. The root does the same things, although not as effectively.

146. Soapwort *(Saponaria officinalis L.), strutium,* no OE word

1. For difficulty in urinating, take the roots of the plant we call *strutium* or . . . [soapwort], and give to eat. It will stimulate the urine.
2. For liver disease, shortness of breath, and for heavy coughing take one spoonful of this plant, pounded; give it to drink in light beer, and it will help. It also heals up any kind of intestinal disturbance and chases out the disease.
3. For bladder stones, take the roots of this same plant, soapwort, or lovage, and of the plant called *capparis* [capers], pound them together and give this to drink in light beer. It soothes the bladder and expels the stones. It also soothes pain in the spleen.

---

246. D'A notes that the name "foxglove" was used throughout the Middle Ages to denote a number of very toxic and powerful plants, among which is modern foxglove (*Digitalis purpurea*), which has the opposite effect from the nightshades. DeV and Hunt also discuss this topic.
247. The Old English original has *leahtras*, diseases or conditions, twice in the sentence. C translates them both as "blotches."

4. For skin irritations, take the same plant, flour, and vinegar. Pound them together and apply them to the irritation. It will clear up.[248]

5. This same plant simmered in wine with barley flour clears up all callouses and infections.

147. Orpine *(Sedum telephium L.), aizon,* no OE word

1. This plant is called *aizon* or . . . [orpine], as though it were everlasting. It has a stem more than a yard long that is the breadth of a finger. It is full of juice and has succulent leaves that are the length of a finger. It grows on hills and sometimes is planted inside a wall.[249] Pounded with flour, this plant helps many diseases of the body, such as sores and rashes and putrefaction and pain, hotness, and burns of the eyes. It helps all these conditions.

2. For headache, take the juice of the same *aizon* [orpine] plant mixed with juice of roses. Apply this to the head, and it relieves the pain.

3. For a bite from a *spalangione* snake, take the same plant and give it to drink in hot wine.

4. Do the same thing for diarrhea, for intestinal worms, and for a bad chill. It cures them up.

148. Sweet Marjoram *(Majorana hortensis), samsuchon, Ellen*[250]

1. For dropsy, take the plant called *sambuscus* or marjoram and give it to drink simmered; it arrests the onset of dropsy. It also helps for inability to urinate and to stimulate the bowels.

2. For carbuncles and for other skin eruptions, take the dried leaves of this same plant, pounded and mixed with honey. Apply this to the sore. It will burst and then heal.

3. For a scorpion's sting, take the same plant, salt, and vinegar; pound them together and make them into a plaster. Apply this to the sting, and it will clear up.

4. For heat and swelling of the eyes, take the same plant mixed with flour and made into a poultice. Smear it on the eyes, and the discomfort will be relieved.

149. French Lavender *(Lavandula stoechas L.), stecas,* no OE name

This plant, which is called *stecas* or . . . [French lavender], has many seeds; they are small and slight, and the plant is like rosemary, except that rosemary has somewhat larger and stiffer leaves.

---

248. C again translates the condition *hreofl* as leprosy, when it appears to be a general skin rash or irritation.

249. Illustrations of early medieval gardens often show many small walled garden plots in which individual kinds of plants are grown. These "walls" are enclosed by a large garden wall.

250. C, DeV = elder *(Sambuscus nigra L.).*

1. Take this plant simmered and give it to drink. It helps chest pain.
2. It is also customary to mix this with many good drinks.

150. Shepherd's Purse *(Capsella bursa-pastoris L.), thyaspis,* no OE name

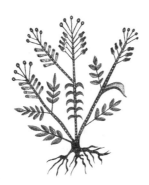

This plant, which is called *thyaspis,* has small, divided leaves one finger in length that incline toward the earth. It has a long, thin stem with purple flowers on the upper part, and its seeds are generated along the entire stem. The whole plant is strong and bitter to the taste. If the juice of this plant is pressed out and a cupful is drunk, all the bitter taste that comes from the bile will be expelled by natural evacuation of the bowels and by expelling vomit.

1. This same plant takes away all painful congestion in the abdomen and it also stimulates a woman's menses.[251]

151. Wood-Sage or Sage-Leaved Germander *(Teucrium scorodonia L.), polios,* no OE word

This plant, which is called *polios* or *omni morbia* or . . . [wood-sage], grows on hills. It sends out many shoots from its roots, and on its upper part, it has seeds like flower heads. It has an unpleasant smell and tastes a little sweet.

1. For snakebite, take the *polis* plant [wood sage] simmered in water and give it to drink. It will heal the bite.

---

251. C translates into Greek the phrase about stimulating the menses.

2. For dropsy, do the same; it relieves the abdomen.
3. For pain of the spleen, take the same plant, simmer it in vinegar, and give to drink. It effectively relieves the pain in the spleen. This same plant strewn or burned in the house chases away snakes. It also heals fresh wounds.

152. St. John's Wort (*Hypericum perforatum L.*), *ypericon*, no OE word

1. This plant, which is called *hypericon* or *corion* because it looks like cumin, has leaves like rue, and many branches grow from one stalk and they are red. It has flowers like a wallflower, and round, somewhat long berries, like barley, on which is the seed, which is dark and smells like wood.[252] It grows in cultivated places. Pounded and drunk, this plant stimulates urination, and it brings on the menses very well if it is laid under the genital organs.[253]
2. For quartan fever, take the same plant, pounded, and give it to drink in wine.
3. For swelling of the shanks of the leg, take the seed of this same plant and give it to drink in wine. Within forty days, the person will be cured.

153. Globe Thistle (*Echinops sphaerocephalus L.*), *acantaleuce*, no OE word

This plant, which is called *acantaleuce* or . . . [globe thistle], grows in stony places and on hills, and it has leaves like wild teasel, but they are softer, whiter and also bushier, and it has a stem more than two yards long and as wide as a finger or a little more.

1. For coughing up blood and for a sore stomach, take the same plant and pound it into powder. Give it to drink in a cupful of water, and it will help.
2. To stimulate the urine, take the same plant pressed of its juice, and give it to drink. It will bring the urine forth.[254]
3. For bad bruises, take the same plant, make it into a poultice, and lay it on the sore; it will purge it. A decoction of this same plant relieves toothache if it is held warm in the mouth.

---

252. *7 þæt sweart 7 on swæce swylce tyrwe.* C = swart and in smack as tar.
253. C writes the word for menses in Greek and calls the genitals "naturalia."
254. The translation of this passage is a particularly good example of Cockayne's style: For stirring of the mie *or urine,* take this same wort, so oozy, pounded, give to drink; it forth leadeth the mie.

4. For cramps, take the seed of this plant, pounded, and give it to drink in water, and it will cure them. The same drink also is of benefit for snakebites.
5. Also, if the plant is worn about the neck, it chases snakes away.

154. Scotch Thistle or Wolly Thistle *(Acanthus mollis), acanton, Beowyrt*

This plant, which is called *acanton* or wolly thistle, grows in pleasant and wet places and sometimes stony ones.

1. To stimulate the intestines and urine, take the dried roots of this same plant made into a powder. Give this to drink in warm water.
2. For lung disease and if any disease settles in the abdomen, if this same plant is eaten, it helps just as we said earlier.

155. Caraway or Cumin *(Carum carvi L.* or *Cuminum cyminum L.),*
quimminon, Cymen

1. For stomachache, take the seed of the plant that is called *quimminon* or cumin simmered in oil and mixed with bran, then simmered together. Make it into a poultice, and put it on the abdomen.
2. For shortness of breath, take the same plant, *quimminon* [cumin], water, and vinegar and mix them together. Give this to drink; it helps effectively. Also, if drunk in wine, it cures snakebite.
3. If the abdomen is tender and hot, take the same plant pounded with grapes or with flour made from beans and make it into a poultice. It will heal the tenderness.
4. It also stops nosebleed when mixed with vinegar.

156. Carline Thistle *(Carlina vulgaris L.), camelleon, Wulfes Tæsl*[255]

This plant, which is called *camelleon alba* or Carline thistle, has rough and thorny leaves, and has in its middle a round and thorny flower head; its flowers are brown, and it has white seeds and white roots with a strong smell.

1. For intestinal worms around the anal region, take the juice from the roots or powder them and give to drink in water in which marjoram or pennyroyal was simmered. It expels the worms plentifully.
2. Five pennies' weight of the root of this same plant taken in wine relieves dropsy, and it has the same strength simmered and drunk for difficulty in urinating.

---

255. C, DeV = Wolf's thistle *(Carlina acaulis).*

157. Artichoke *(Scolymus maculatus* or *S. Hispanicus L.), scolymbus,* no OE word[256]

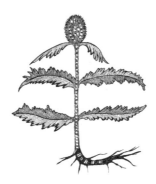

1. This plant, called *scolimbos* or . . . [artichoke]: simmered in wine and drunk removes the bad smell from armpits and the rest of the body.
2. This same plant cures bad-smelling urine and provides healing food for people.

158. German Iris or Blue Iris *(Iris spp. L* or *germanica L.), iris Illyrica,* no OE word

This plant, called *iris Illyrica* or . . . [German iris], has this name for the diversity of its blossoms, because it is thought that it resembles the rainbow in the sky in color. It is called *iris* in Latin, and it grows best and strongest in Illyrica. It has leaves like sea onion or squill, which the Greeks call *xifian,* and it has strong roots with a strong odor. It should be folded up in a linen cloth and hung in the shade so that it can thoroughly dry, because its nature is hot and soporific.

1. For deep coughs that the person cannot clear away because they are thick and soft, take ten pennies' weight of the finely pounded and powdered root of this plant and give it to drink in light beer on an empty stomach: four cups for three days or until the cough clears up.

    In the same way, the powder of this same plant taken in light beer induces sleep and relieves abdominal discomfort.

---

256. DeV = artichoke *(Scolymus cardunculus L.).*

2. In the same way, the powder of this same plant heals snakebites. The same quantity of the powder of this plant, as we said before, mixed with vinegar and drunk benefits him[257] whose semen spontaneously ejects—the condition the Greeks call gonorrhea. Indeed, if the same quantity is mixed with wine, it will stimulate the menses even though they have been gone for some time.

3. For hard swellings and pimples, take the whole root of this plant dried thoroughly and then soaked. Pound it then to make it soft and make it into a poultice. Put it on the sore, and it will disperse.

4. It also helps a headache when mixed with vinegar and juice of roses.

159. Sea Onion, Squill *(Urginea maritima L.), eleborum album,* no OE name[258]

1. For liver disease, take the plant *eleborum album* or . . . [squill], dried and pounded into powder. Give it to drink in warm water, six spoonfuls of the powder. It will heal the liver. The same thing helps against all poisons when taken in wine.

160. Larkspur *(Delphinium Ajacis L.), delfinion,* no OE word

1. For quartan fever, take the juice of the plant called *delfinion,* carefully gathered and pounded and mixed with pepper. There should be an odd number of peppercorns, that is, from the first day, thirty one, and the next day, seventeen, and the third day thirteen. If you give this before the onset of the fever, relief will be experienced very quickly.

161. Viper's Bugloss *(Echium plantagineum* or *vulgare L.), aecios,* no OE word

This plant, called *æcios* or . . . [viper's bugloss], has seeds that look like a snake's head and long, stiff leaves, and it sends out many stems. It has thin, somewhat thorny leaves and brown flowers between the leaves. Between the flowers, it has, as we said before, seeds that look like a snake's head. Its root is small and dark.

1. For snakebite, take the root of this same *aecios* plant [viper's bugloss] and give it to drink in wine. It helps both before and after the bite. The same drink also relieves pain in the loins, and the dried

257. At this point, C translates the rest of the passage into Latin, with the words for gonorrhea and menses given in Greek. As noted earlier, according to Riddle, *Contraception and Abortion,* the latter part of the remedy might have been a method of abortion.

258. DeV and D'A note that no such herb or remedy are found in any edition of *De herbis feminis. A Scilla* is also given in chapter 43. For more on this plant, see Jerry Stannard, "Squill in Ancient and Medieval Materia Medica," in Jerry Stannard, *Pristina Medicamenta: Ancient and Medieval Medical Botany* (London: Ashgate Variorum, 1999).

plant stimulates breast milk. Truly, there is power in the plant, its root and its seeds.

162. Moneywort *(Lysimachia nummularia L.), centimorbia,* no OE word

1. This plant, *centimorbia* or . . . [moneywort], grows in cultivated places, in stony places, on hills and in pleasant places. From one piece of turf it sends out many shoots. It has small, round, divided leaves, and it has the power to cure. If a horse is injured on the back or on the shoulder, take this plant, thoroughly dried and pounded into powder, sprinkle it onto the sore and the plant will heal it. You will be surprised at its effectiveness.

163. Water germander or barrenwort *(Epimedium alpinum L.* or t*eucrium scordium L.), scordias,* no OE word

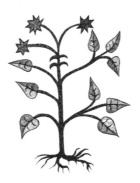

This plant, *scordias* or . . . [water germander], smells like a leek and because of this is called *scordios.* This plant grows on the moors and it has round leaves that are bitter to the taste. It has a four-edged stem and reddish-yellow flowers.

1. To stimulate the urine, take the fresh, pounded *scordios* plant [water germander] eaten in wine or the dried plant simmered in wine. Give this latter to drink, and it will stimulate urination.
2. The same thing benefits snakebite, all poisons, and stomachache, and as we said before, helps difficulty in urinating.
3. For formation of phlegm in the chest,[259] take ten pennies' weight of the same plant mixed with honey. Give one spoonful to eat, and the chest will be purged.

---

259. *Wið þæs gerynnincge þæs worsmes ym ðs breost.* C = For the running of ratten about the breasts. I think the chest is intended instead of the breasts; the Latin original in DeV is fragmentary, but manuscript O lists this remedy *Ad pectus.*

4. For gout, take the same plant pounded into vinegar or water. Give it to drink, and it will help.
5. For fresh wounds, take the same plant, pounded, and smear it on the wound. It will heal them. Also, mixed with honey it purges and heals old wounds, and powdered, it inhibits skin from growing.

164. Bishop's-Weed *(Ammi maius), ami,* no OE word

1. This plant, called *ami* or *miluium* or . . . [bishop's-weed], has seed that is given in wine and is good for medications. It is beneficial for abdominal discomfort, for difficulty in urinating, and for bites of wild animals. It also brings on the menses.[260] For blemishes on the body, the seed of this same plant pounded in honey clears up the blemishes.
2. For paleness and discoloration of the body, the same: that is, that you apply the same thing to the body, or drink it, and it will take the discoloration away.

165. Wallflower *(Cheiranthus cheiri L.), uiola, Banwyrt*[261]

This plant, called *uiola* or wallflower, comes in three varieties: one is dark purple, one white, and the third is yellow. The yellow one, however, is best suited for medications.

1. For pain and inflammation of the womb, pound the same plant and put it under the woman; it will help. It also brings on menstruation.[262]
2. For various disorders of the rectum, called *ragadas*, that is primarily for a discharge of blood, take the pounded leaves of this same plant and make them into a poultice. It heals all of the disorders.
3. The leaves of this same plant pounded and mixed with honey heal canker sores of the teeth, from which the teeth often fall out.
4. To stimulate menstruation, take ten pennies' weight of the seeds of this plant, either pounded and drunk in wine, or mixed with honey and put on the sexual organ. It brings about menstruation and takes the fetus from the womb.[263]
5. For pain of the spleen, take the roots of this same plant pounded in vinegar. Lay it on the spleen and it will be of benefit.

---

260. C gives menses in Greek.
261. DeV and Bierbaumer = wild pansy *(Viola tricolor L.)*.
262. C gives only Greek terms for womb and menstruation.
263. All the references to menstruation and to what this remedy is used for are in Greek in C. This is clearly an abortifacient.

166. Sweet Violet *(Viola odorata L.)*, *uiola purpurea*, no OE word

1. For fresh wounds or old ones, take the leaves of the *uiola purpurea* plant [violet] and lard in equal quantities. Apply this to the wound, and it will effectively heal it. It also reduces swellings and callouses.
2. For constipation, take the flowers of this same plant mixed with honey and soaked in very good wine. The constipation will be relieved.

167. Unidentified

This plant, called *zamalentition* or . . . , grows in stony places and on hills.

1. For all wounds, take the *zamaltentition* plant powdered thoroughly in unsalted lard, and smear it on the wound. All will be healed.
2. For ulcerous sores, take the dried plant and pounded into a fine powder. Apply this to the wound, and it will purge the pain from the sores.

168. Alkanet *(Anchusa tinctoria L.)*, *ancusa*, no OE name

This plant, called *ancusa* or . . . [alkanet], grows in cultivated places and on smooth ones. You should pick it in the month of March. There are two varieties of this plant: one the Africans call *barbatus* or bearded. The other is very good for medications, and it was originally grown in Persia. It has sharp, thorny leaves without stalks.

1. For a bad burn, take the roots of the *ancusa* [alkanet] plant soaked in oil and then mixed with wax like you would make a plaster or poultice. Apply this to the burns, and it will heal them in a wonderful manner.

169. Fleawort or Fleaseed *(Plantago psyllium L.)*, *psillios, Coliandre*[264]

This plant is called *psillos* because it has seeds like fleas, and for this reason, it is *pulicaris* in Latin. It has small, hairy leaves, and its stem is bushy with branches. It is by nature dry and weak, and it grows in cultivated places.

1. For hard swellings and other swellings, take the seeds of this plant pounded in one oil jar plus two cups of water, and mix them together. Give this to drink. Take some of the same seeds, make them into a plaster, put them on the sore, and it will be healed.
2. For a headache, take the same with juice of roses soaked in water.

---

264. D'A notes that the plant illustrated in the MS is coriander, as its caption indicates, but that the remedies describe uses for *psyllium*—however the confusion began centuries before. All the Latin versions and all the extant mss of *De herbis femininis* make the same mistake. C translates it as coriander, but notes the confusion over what it is.

170. Sweet Briar, Eglantine *(Rosa canina* or *rubiginosa L.),* no OE word

This plant, called *cynosbatus* or . . . [sweet briar], when it is picked from its stem, is harsh on the throat and disagreeable before meals, but nevertheless, it will purge the chest, and anything sour or bitter; although it harms the stomach, it benefits the spleen greatly. If the flowers of this plant are drunk, they affect a person in a way so that the intestines and urine will take out disease. It also purifies bleeding.

1. Again, for pain of the spleen, take the well-cleaned bark from the root of this plant and lay it on the spleen. It will be useful and beneficial. The person who undergoes this treatment should lie facing up lest he feel impatient about the strength of this treatment.[265]

171. Peony *(Paeonia L.), aglaofotis,* no OE name[266]

This plant, called *aglaofotis* or . . . [peony], shines at night like a lamp and it helps with many diseases.

1. For tertian or quartan fever, take the juice of this same plant mixed with oil of roses. Smear it on the sick person; undoubtedly you will help the person.
2. If anyone suffers a storm while rowing, take the same plant and set it on fire for incense; the storm will be held back.
3. For cramps and tremors, take the same plant and keep it with you. If a person carries some with him, evil will be afraid.

172. Caper *(Capparis spinosa L.), Capparis, Wudubend*

1. For pain of the spleen, take the root of the plant called *capparis* [caper], pound it into powder and make it into a poultice. Apply this to the spleen, and it will dry it up. But yet, fasten the person, lest he shake the medication off him because of the pain. After three hours, lead the person to the bath, bathe him well, and he will be relieved.

173. Eryngo *(Eryngium supp.), eringius,* no OE word[267]

This plant, called *eringius* or . . . [eryngo], has soft leaves when it first grows, and they are sweet to the taste, and one eats them as other plants. After that, they are sharp and thorny, and it has white or green stalks, on the upper part,

---

265. DeV notes about the last statement that the Anglo-Saxon translator missed the meaning of the Latin, which reads "lest, being unable to endure the potency of the medicine, he should scatter the remedy."
266. DeV says this is sunflower *(Helianthus annuus L.),* C calls it peony, but of another variety. DeV notes that this chapter is not found in any of the Latin texts he consulted.
267. DeV = sea holly *(eryngium maritmum L.).*

from which grow sharp, thorny prickles. It has a long root, its outer part is black, and it has a good smell. This plant grows in fields and in rough places.

1. To stimulate urination, take the plant called *eringius* [eryngo] pounded and give it to drink in wine. It will not only stimulate urination, but also the menses and bowel movement, and it reduces swellings. In addition, it benefits liver disease and snake bites.
2. The same eaten with the seeds of what is called the *olisatra* [Alexanders or horse parsley] plant also benefits many diseases of the abdomen.
3. For swelling of the breasts, take the same plant made into a poultice, and put it on the breasts. It will dispel all the diseased matter from the breasts.
4. For sting of a scorpion and for all bites from snakes and mad dogs, take the same plant and make it into a plaster. Put it on the wound (the wound is first opened with an iron tool); it is laid on it so that the sick person does not perceive the smell. Prepared the same way, this same plant greatly benefits skin diseases, and it also relieves gout if one puts it on at the onset.

174. Cleavers, Goosegrass *(Galium aparine L.), philantropos, Clate*

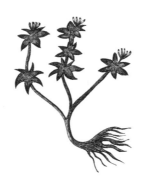

This plant is called *philantropos*—or in our language "loving people"—because it willingly adheres to people, and it has seeds like a human navel. It is also called cleavers. It sends out many branches that are long and four-sided, and its leaves are stiff. Its has big stems and white flowers and seeds that are hard, round, and hollow in the middle, and, as we said before, they look like a human navel.[268]

_____

268. C seems to have skipped over some of the Old English. He has ". . . it is stiff in leaves, and it hath a great stalk, and in the middle is hollow, as we before said, in the manner in which a mans navel is."

1. For bites from a snakes and from the *spalangione* spider, take the juice of this plant mixed in wine. Give it to drink, and it will be of benefit.
2. For earache, take the juice of this same plant, drip it into the ear, and it will relieve the pain.

175. Yarrow *(Achillea spp.), achillea,* no OE word[269]

The *achillea* or . . . [yarrow] plant grows in cultivated soil and near water; it has yellow and white flowers.

1. For fresh wounds, take the pounded flower heads of this plant and lay them on the wound. They will take away the pain, will heal the wound, and stop the bleeding.
2. If a woman is troubled by fluid flowing from her sexual organ, take the same plant, soaked, and lay it beneath the woman, who is seated. It takes away all the smell of the fluid from her.[270]
3. Also this same plant drunk in water relieves diarrhea very well.

This plant is called "achillea" because it is said that Lord Achilles used it often to treat wounds.

176. Castor-Oil Plant *(Ricinus communis L.), ricinus,* no OE word

1. To turn away hail and storms, if you have the *ricinus*[271] or . . . [castor-oil plant] in your possession or you hang its seeds in your house or have it or its seeds in some place, it will turn back a hail storm. If you hang it or its seeds aboard ship, it is surprising how it appeases all storms. You must pick this plant while saying this: *Herba ricinum, precor uti adsis meis incantationibus et auertas grandines, fulgora, et omnes tempestates, per nomen omnipotentis Dei qui te iussit nasci.* That is in our language: Ricinum plant, I ask that you be present at my song and that you turn away the hail and lightning flashes and every storm, through the name of almighty God, who caused you to be made.

Also, you must be clean when you pick the plant.

---

269. DeV has sneezewort *(Achillea ptarmica L.).*
270. C translates the whole entry into Latin. His Latin translation and the supposed Latin original as given in DeV do not read the same. The Latin is talking about heavy menstruation, whereas the Old English original does not say this is specifically menstrual *(monaðlic)* flux; from the Old English, it could be merely a discharge.
271. This plant is not in any Latin text, according to DeV. For some reason, C adds in italics after the name of the plant, "and which is not a native of England."

177. Black Horehound *(Ballota nigra L.), polloten,* no OE name

This plant, called *polloten* or *porrum nigrum* or . . . [black horehound], has thorny, dark, rough stems and broader leaves than a leek but darker. They have a strong smell, and its power is sharp.

1.   For dog bite, take the leaves of this plant pounded with salt. Lay this on the wound, and it will heal it in a wonderful manner.
2.   Again, for wounds, take the leaves of this plant pounded with honey and lay them on the wound. It will heal each wound.

178. Nettle *(Urtica dioica L.), urtica, Netele*

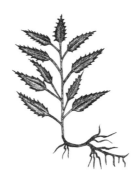

1.   For wounds that have cooled, take the juice of this same plant, called *urtica* or nettle, mixed with the sediment from oil with a little salt added, and put it on the wound. Within three days it will be healed.
2.   For swellings, do the same thing, that is, put it on the swelling in the same manner, and it will be healed.
3.   If any part of the body has been struck, take the same plant, pounded, and lay it on the wound. It will be healed.
4.   For pain in the loins, if they are injured because something happened to them or because of a chill or anything else, take the juice of this plant and oil in equal quantities and simmer them together. Put this on where it hurts the most, and within three days you will heal the person.
5.   For foul, putrefied wounds, take the same plant pounded and add a little salt. Fasten this to the wound, and within three days it will be healthy.
6.   For a woman's menses, take the same plant, pounded thoroughly in a mortar so that it is very soft. Add to it a little honey, take some moist wool that has been teased, and then use it to smear the genitals with

the medication. Then give it to the woman, so that she can lay it under her. That same day, it will stop the bleeding.[272]

7. So that the cold will not bother you, take the same plant soaked in oil and rub it on the hands and all over the body. You will not experience cold on any of your body.

179. Greater Periwinkle *(Vinca maior L.), priapisci,* no OE word

1. This plant, called *priapisci* or *uicaperuica,* is beneficial against many things, but first against the onset of being possessed,[273] then against snakes, wild animals, poison, any threat, envy, and terror. It is also beneficial so that you will obtain grace. If you have this plant with you, you are happy and always contented. You must pick the plant saying the following: *Te precor uicaperuica multis utilitatibus habenda ut uenias ad me hilaris florens cum tuis uirtutibus, ut ea mihi prestes, ut tutus et felix sim semper a uenenis et ab iracundia inlesus.* This is in our language: I pray you, periwinkle, you who has many uses, that you gladly come to me with your powers blooming, that you make me so that I will be protected and always happy and not harmed by poison and by anger.

When you want to pick the plant, you should be free from any kind of uncleanliness. You must pick it when the moon is nine nights old, and eleven nights, thirteen nights, thirty nights, and when it is one night old.

180. Common Gromwell *(Lithospermum officinale L.), lithospermon, Sunnancorn*

This plant, called *lithospermon* or . . . [common gromwell], grows in Italy, originally in Crete, and it has larger leaves than rue and straight. At its top it has white, round stones, like pearls, the size of peas, and they are as hard as pearls, and also bunched together. They are hollow inside and the seeds are inside.

1. For bladder stones and for difficulty in urinating, take five pennies' weight of these stones [from the plant] and give them to drink in wine. It will break up the bladder stones and lead forth the urine.

---

272. C translates the entire passage into Latin.
273. Literally, possessed by demons.

181. Stavisacre or Lousewort *(Dephinium stafisagria L.), stauisagria,* no
OE word

The plant called *stauis agria* or . . . [lousewort] has leaves like a grape and a
straight stem, and it has seeds in green pods the size of peas. It is triangular
and sour and dark, but it is white inside and bitter to the taste.

1. For general bodily discomfort,[274] take fifteen seeds of this plant
    pounded in light beer. Give it to drink, and it purges the body by
    vomiting. After the person has drunk the drink, he should walk
    around and get the circulation going before he vomits. When the per-
    son begins to vomit, he should ingest light beer often, lest the power
    of the plant burn the throat and choke him.
2. For scaly skin or scabs, take the seeds of this same plant and roses
    and pound them together. Smear it on the dry places, and they will
    heal.
3. For toothache and sore gums, take the seeds of this same plant and
    simmer them in vinegar. Hold some of the vinegar in the mouth for
    quite a while. It will cure the toothache, sore gums, and all putrefac-
    tion in the mouth.

182. No English name *(Eryngium campestre L.), gorgonion,* no OE word[275]

1. This plant, called *gorgonion* or . . . , grows in shady places and wet
    ones. About this plant it is said that its root looks like the head of a
    snake that is called a gorgon, and that the branches, so it is also said,
    have the color, the eyes, and nose of snakes.
2. This root makes any person like itself, whether the color of gold or of
    silver. If you want to pick the plant with its roots, be careful that the
    sun does not shine on it, lest its color and strength be changed by the
    sun's brightness. Cut it only with a curved and very hard iron tool;
    and whoever intends to cut it must turn away from it because it is not
    permitted that anyone see its entire root. Whoever has this root with
    him will avoid all evil footprints coming toward him; indeed,
    because of it, the evil person will either turn away or yield to him.

183. Melilot *(Melilotus officinalis L.), milotis,* no OE word

1. This plant, which is called *milotis* or . . . [melilot], grows in culti-
    vated places and wet ones. You should pick this plant when the moon

---

274. *yfelan wætan.* C = evil humours. In view of the remedy, it seems to be general fever and
being sick to the stomach.
275. D'A lists this plant as unidentified. C, DeV, Bierbaumer = field eryngo.

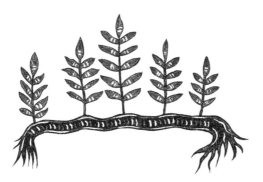

is on the wane, in the month of August. Take the root of this plant, fasten it to a weaving thread, and hang it around your neck. During that year, you will not have dim eyes, or if it has already happened to you, it will quickly disappear, and you will be healthy. This remedy is tested.

2. For muscle spasms, take the juice of this same plant, rub it on, and the condtion will abate. Also, it is said about this plant that it flowers twice a year.

184. Tassel Hyacinth *(Muscari comosum Mill.), bulbus,* no OE word[276]

This plant, called *bulbus* or . . . [tassel hyacinth], has two varieties: one is red and beneficial for stomach pain, the other is bitter to the taste, is called *scillodes,* and is also beneficial for the stomach. Both are powerful, and when eaten as food, strengthen the body.

1. For swellings and gout and for any injury, take this plant pounded by itself or mixed with honey. Put it on the soreness as needed.
2. For dropsy, take this same plant, as we said before, pounded, and lay it on the abdomen. Mixed with honey, it also cures dog bites. If it is mixed with pepper and applied, it stops a person from sweating. It also lessens stomach pain.
3. For sores that come of themselves, take the root of this plant pounded with oil, hot flour-meal, and soap, as you would make a poultice, and lay it on the sores. It also cures the disease the Greeks call *hostopyturas*, that is dandruff, and also what they call *achoras*, or scabies, which very often makes the hair fall out. In addition, it rids the face of pimples when pounded with vinegar or honey.
4. Also, taken with vinegar, it heals swelling and ruptures in the abdomen.

276. DeV = onion *(Allium cepa L.).*

About this plant, it is said that it is supposed to grow in dragon's blood at the top of mountains in thick groves.

185. Bitter Cucumber *(Citrullus colocynthis), colocynthisagria,* no OE word[277]

This plant, called *colocynthisagria* or *curcurbita agrestis* or *frigilla* [bitter cucumber], just like other gourds expands its branches over the ground. It has divided leaves like a cucumber and round and bitter fruit. It should be picked at the time just as its green gives way to yellow.

1. To move the bowels, take two pennies' weight of the tender inside of the fruit without the seeds pounded in light beer. Give this to drink. It will move the bowels.

---

277. DeV = *Cucumis colocynthis.* This is the only chapter that does not begin with a painting of the plant.

References

Ackerknecht, Erwin H. *A Short History of Medicine.* New York: The Ronald Press, 1955.

André, J. *Lexique des termes de botanique en latin.* Paris: Klincksieck, 1956.

"Anglo-Saxon Leechdoms: Medicine and Astronomy in the Dark Ages." *Dublin University Magazine* 69 (May 1867).

Anglo-Saxon Manuscripts in Microfiche Facsimile (Binghamton, NY: Medieval & Renaissance Texts & Studies, 1994).

Arber, Agnes. *Herbals: Their Origin and Evolution, A Chapter in the History of Botany, 1470–1670.* Cambridge: Cambridge University Press, 1938.

Arnold, Matthew. "On Translating Homer." In *On Translating Homer: With F. W Newman's "Homeric Translation" and Arnold's "Last Words."* London: Routledge, n.d.

Baring-Gould, Sabine. *Early Reminiscences: 1834–1864.* New York: E. P. Dutton & Co., 1922.

Bartrip, Peter. "Secret Remedies, Medical Ethics, and the Finances of the British Medical Journal." In Robert Baker, ed., *The Codification of Medical Morality: Historical and Philosophical Studies of the Formalization of Western Medical Morality in the Eighteenth and Nineteenth Centuries*, Vol. 2. Dordrecht: Kluwer Academic Publishers, 1995.

Bately, J. M. "Old English Prose Before and During the Reign of Alfred." *Anglo-Saxon England* 17 (1988): 93–138.

———. "The Literary Prose of King Alfred's Reign: Translation or Transformation?" Inaugural Lecture in the Chair of English and Medieval Literature delivered at University of London King's College on 4 March 1980.

Beccaria, Augusto. *I Codici di Medicina del Periodo Presalernitano (Secoli Ix, X e XI)*. Roma: Edisioni de Storia e Letteratura, 1956.

Bennett, J. M., E. A. Clark, J. F. O'Barr, B. A. Vilen, and S. Westphal-Wihl, eds. *Sisters and Workers in the Middle Ages*. Chicago: University of Chicago Press, 1989.

Berberich, Hugo, ed. *Das Herbarium Apulei nach einer frühmittelenglischen Fassung*. 1901. Reprint. Amsterdam: Swets und Zeitlinger NV Nachgedruckt, 1966.

Bierbaumer, Peter. *Der Botanische Wortschatz des Altenglischen*. 3 vols. Frankfurt: Peter Lang, 1975.

Blair, Peter Hunter. *An Introduction to Anglo-Saxon England*. Cambridge: Cambridge University Press, 1959.

Bloc, Marc. *The Royal Touch: Sacred Monarchy and Scrofula in England and France*. Translated by J. E. Anderson. London: Routledge and Keegan, 1973.

Bloomfield, Josephine Helm. "Diminished by Kindness: Frederick Klaeber's Rewriting of Wealhtheow." *Journal of English and Germanic Philology* 93 (April 1994): 183–203.

——— . "The Canonization of Editorial Sensibility in Beowulf: A Philological and Historical Reassessment of Klaeber's Edition." Ph.D. diss., University of California at Davis, 1991.

Blunt, Wilfrid and Sandra Raphael. *The Illustrated Herbal*. New York: Thames and Hudson, 1979.

Bolton, W. F. *A Living Language: The History and Structure of English*. New York: Random House, 1982.

Bonser, Wilifrid. *The Medical Background of the Anglo-Saxons: A Study in History, Psychology, and Folklore*. London: The Wellcome Historical Medical Library, 1963.

Bosworth, Joseph. *The Origin of the Germanic and Scandinavian Languages and Nations: with a Sketch of their Literature, and short chronological specimens of the Anglo-Saxon, Friesic, Flemish, Dutch, the German from the Meso-Goths to the Present Time, the Icelandic, Danish, Norwegian, and Swedish: Tracing the Progress of these Languages and their Connection with the Anglo-Saxon and the Present English*. London: Longman, 1836.

———. *Latin Construing: or Easy and Progressive Lessons for Classical Authors, with Rules for Translating Latin into English*. London: W. Simpkin and H. Marshall, 1824.

————. *Elements of Anglo-Saxon Grammar*. London: Richard Taylor, 1823.

Brewer, Charlotte. "Walter William Skeat." In Helen Damico, ed. *Medieval Scholarship: Biographical Studies on the Formation of a Discipline*. New York: Garland Publishing, 1998.

Brodin, Gösta. *Agnus Castus, A Middle English Herbal, reconstructed from various manuscripts*. Uppsala: Lundequistska, 1950.

Brown, Peter. *The World of Late Antiquity*. London: Harcourt Brace Jovanovich, 1971.

Burke, James T. *This Miserable Kingdom: The Story of the Spanish Presence in New Mexico and the Southwest from the Beginning until the 18th Century*. Santa Fe, NM: Christo Rey Church, 1973.

Cameron, M. L. "Anglo-Saxon Medicine and Magic." In *Anglo-Saxon England* 17 (1988): 191–215.

————. "The Sources of Medical Knowledge in Anglo-Saxon England." In *Anglo-Saxon England* 11 (1983): 135–55.

Campbell, Sheila, Bert Hall, David Klausner, eds. *Health, Disease and Healing in Medieval Culture*. New York: St. Martin's Press, 1992.

Cantor, Norman. *The Civilization of the Middle Ages*. 1963. Reprint. New York: HarperCollins, 1993.

Cockayne, Oswald. *The Shrine: a Collection of Occasional Papers on Dry Subjects*. London: Williams and Northgate, 1870.

————. "Mr. Cockayne's Narrative." Privately printed 1869. Archives of King's College School.

————, ed. *Hali Meidenhad: An Alliterative Homily of the Thirteenth Century*. London: Trübner and Co., 1866.

————, ed. *Leechdoms, Wortcunning, and Starcraft of Early England*. 1864. 3 vols., Rolls Series, Vol. 35. Reprint. London: Kraus Reprint Ltd., 1965.

————, ed. *Leechdoms, Wortcunning, and Starcraft of Early England*. 1864. 3 vols., Rolls Series, Vol. 35. Reprint. Introduction by Charles Singer. London: The Holland Press, 1961.

————. *Seinte Marherete: The Meiden ant Martyr*. 1862. London: Trübner and Co., 1866.

————. *Narratiunculae Anglice Conscriptae: De Pergamenis Exscribebat Notis Illustrabat Eruditis Copiam*. London: Iohannem R. Smith, 1861.

————— . *Spoon and Sparrow, ΣΠΕΝΔΕΙΝ AND ΨΑΡ, FUNDERE AND PASSER; or, English Roots in the Greek, Latin, and Hebrew: Being a consideration of the Affinities of the Old English, Anglo-Saxon, or Teutonic Portion of our Tongue to the Latin and Greek; with a few pages on the Relation of the Hebrew to the European Languages.* London: Parker, Son, and Bourn, 1861.

————— . *The Civil History of the Jews from Joshua to Hadrian; with a Preliminary Chapter on the Mosaic History.* London: John W. Parker, West Strand, 1845.

Cockayne, Oswald and Edmund Brock, eds. *þe Liflade of St. Juliana: From Two Old English Manuscripts of 1230 A.D.* London: Trübner and Co., 1872.

Collins, Minta. *Medieval Herbals: The Illustrative Tradition.* London: British Library, 2000.

Copeland, Rita. *Rhetoric, Hermenutics, and Translation in the Middle Ages: Academic traditions and vernacular texts.* Cambridge: Cambridge University Press, 1991.

Cornish Telegraph. "Identification of the gentleman supposed to have committed suicide at St. Ives." 25 June 1873.

Cornish Telegraph. "Discovery of the body of a traveller who had committed suicide a fortnight since." 18 June 1873.

Crawford, Amanda McQuade. "Western Herbal History." Albuquerque, NM: The National College of Phytotherapy, 1996.

Crosby, Alfred W., Jr. *The Columbian Exchange: Biological and Cultural Consequences of 1492.* Westport, CT: Greenwood Publishing Co., 1972.

Culpepper, Nicholas. *Culpepper's Herbal,* ed. David Potterton. New York: Sterling Publishing Co., 1983.

Curtin, L. S. M. *Healing Herbs of the Upper Rio Grande.* Los Angeles: Southwest Museum, 1965.

Damico, Helen, ed. *Medieval Scholarship: Biographical Studies on the Formation of a Discipline.* Vol. 2. New York: Garland Press, 1998.

D'Aronco, M. A. "The Old English Herbal: a proposed dating for the translation." University of Udine, Italy, 1998.

————— . "The botanical lexicon of the Old English Herbarium." In *Anglo-Saxon England* 17 (1988): 15–33.

D'Aronco, M. A. and M. L. Cameron. *The Old English Illustrated Pharmacopoeia.* Copenhagen: Rosenkilde and Bagger, 1998; published as "L'erbaeio anglosassone, un' ipotesi sulla data della traduzione," *Romanobarborica* 13 (1995, pub. 1996): 325–365.

De Vriend, Hubert Jan. *The Old English Herbarium and Medicina de Quadrupedibus.* Early English Text Society. O.S. 286. London: Oxford University Press, 1984.

Deegan, Marilyn. "A Critical Edition of MS. B. L. Royal 12. D. XVII: Bald's 'Leechbook' Vols. 1 and 2." Ph.D. diss., University of Manchester, 1988.

Deegan, Marilyn and D. G. Scragg. *Medicine in Early Medieval England.* Manchester: University of Manchester, 1989.

Faulkner, Peter, ed. *William Morris: The Cultural Heritage.* London: Routledge and Kegan Paul, 1973.

Fitoterapia. Indena Company, Italy. http://www.idena.it/fitoterapia.

Frantzen, Allen J. *Desire for Origins: New Language, Old English, and Teaching the Tradition.* New Brunswick: Rutgers University Press, 1990.

Frantzen, Allen J. and John D. Niles. *Anglo-Saxonism and the Construction of Social Identity.* Gainesville: University Press of Florida, 1997.

Frazer, James G. *The Golden Bough.* New York: The MacMillan Company, 1940.

Getz, Faye. *Medicine in the English Middle Ages.* Princeton: Princeton University Press, 1998.

Gilligham, R. G. "An Edition of Abbot Aelfric's Old English-Latin Glossary with Commentary." Ph.D. diss., Ohio State University, 1981.

Grape-Albers, Heide. *Medicina Antiqua: Codex Vindobonensis 93.* Introduction by Peter Murray Jones. London: Harvey Miller, 1999.

—————. *Spätantike Bilder aus der Welt des Arztes: Medizinische Bilderhandschriften der Spätantike und Ihre Mittelalterliche Überliferund.* Wiesbaden: Guido Pressler Verlag, 1977.

Grattan, J. H. G. and Charles Singer. *Anglo-Saxon Magic and Medicine.* London: Oxford University Press, 1952.

Green, Monica. *The Trotula: A Medieval Compendium of Women's Medicine.* Philadelphia: University of Pennsylvania Press, 2001.

—————. "Women's Medical Practice and Health Care in Medieval Europe." In J. M. Bennett, E. A. Clark, J. F. O'Barr, B. A. Vilen, and S. Westphal-Wihl. *Sisters and Workers in the Middle Ages.* Chicago: University of Chicago Press, 1989.

Gross, Arthur. "Wolframs Schlangenliste (*Parzifal* 481) und Pseudo-Apuleius." In *Licht der Natur: Medizin in Fachliteratur und Dichtung*, eds. J. Domes, W. Gerabek, B. Haage, C. Weißer and V. Zimmermann. Göppingen: Kümmerle Verlag, 1994.

Grieve, M. *A Modern Herbal*. 1931. Reprint. New York: Dover Publications, 1971.

Gunther, Robert T. ed. *The Greek Herbal of Dioscorides*. 1934. Reprint. London: Hafner Publishing Co., 1968.

Guyonvarc'h, Christian-J. *Magie, médecine et divination chez les Celtes*. Paris: Payot, 1997.

Hadfield, Miles. *Gardens in Britain*. London: Hutchinson, 1960.

Hall, J. R. "William G. Medlicott (1816–1883): An American Book Collector and His Collection." *Harvard Library Bulletin*, n.s., 1:1 (Spring 1990): 13–46.

Hankins, Freda Richards. "*Bald's Leechbook* Reconsidered." Ph.D. diss., University of North Carolina at Chapel Hill, 1991.

Harvey, John. *Medieval Gardens*. London: B. T. Batsford, 1981.

Hilbelink, Aaltje Johanna Geertruida. *Cotton MS Vitellius C. iii of the Herbarium Apulei*. Amsterdam: NV Swets und Zeitlanger, 1930.

Hofstetter, W. "Zur lateinischen Quellen des altenglischen Pseudo-Dioskurides." *Anglia* 101 (1983): 315–60.

Holland, Bart K., ed. *Prospecting for Drugs in Ancient and Medieval European Texts: A Scientific Approach*. Amsterdam: Harwood Academic Publishers, 1996.

———. "Prospecting for drugs in ancient texts," *Nature* 369 (30 June 1994): 701–2.

Hollis, Stephanie and Michael Wright. *Old English Prose of Secular Learning*. Cambridge: D. S. Brewer, 1992.

Howald, Ernst and H. E. Sigerist. *Antonii Musae de Herba Vettonica Liber, Pseudo-Apulei Herbarius, Anonymi de Taxone Liber, etc.* In *Corpus Medicorum Latinorum*. Vol. 4. Leipzig, 1927.

Hunger, F. W. T. *The Herbal of Apuleius*. Leiden: Brill, 1936.

Hunt, Thurman. "From Plant Lore to Pharmacy." In Holland, Bart K., ed. *Prospecting for Drugs in Ancient and Medieval European Texts: A Scientific Approach*. Amsterdam: Harwood Academic Publishers, 1996.

Hunt, Tony. *Plant Names of Medieval England*. Cambridge: D. S. Brewer, 1989.

Inglis, Brian. *A History of Medicine*. Cleveland: The World Publishing Company, 1965.

Jansen-Sieben, ed., *Artes Mechanicae en Europe médiévale/en middeleeuws Europa*. Bruxelles: Archives et Bibliothèques de Belgique, 1989.

Jenkins, Myra Ellen and Albert H. Schroeder. *A Brief History of New Mexico*. Albuquerque: University of New Mexico Press, 1974.

Jolly, Karen Louise. *Popular Religion in Late Saxon England: Elf Charms in Context*. Chapel Hill: University of North Carolina Press, 1996.

Jones, Peter Murray. *Medieval Medicine in Illuminated Manuscripts*. London: British Library, 1998.

Keil, Gundolf. *Fachprosa-Studien: Beiträge zur mittelalterlichen Wissenschafts- und Geistesgeschichte*. Berlin: E. Schmidt, 1982.

Keil, Gundolf and Paul Schnitzer, eds. *Das Lorscher Arzneibuch und die Frühmittelalterliche Medizin: Verhandlungen des Medizinhistorischen Symposiums im September 1989 in Lorsch*. Lorsch: Verlag Laurissa, 1991.

Ker, Neil R. *Catalogue of Manuscripts Containing Anglo-Saxon*. Oxford: Clarendon Press, 1957.

Keys, Thomas E. *The History of Surgical Anesthesia*. 1945. New York: Dover Publications, 1963.

Kristeller, P. O. "The School of Salerno." *Bulletin of the History of Medicine* 17 (1945): 138–94.

Lawrence, George H. M. "Herbals: Their History and Significance." In George H. M. Lawrence and Kenneth F. Baker, *History of Botany*. Los Angeles: University of California and the Hunt Botanical Library, 1965.

London Times. 25 June 1873. Obituary Column. "T. O. Cockayne."

Lye, Edward. *Dictionarium saxonico et gothico-latinum,* ed. O. Manning. London: B. White, 1772.

M. S. Cotton Vitellius C. iii. In *Anglo-Saxon Manuscripts in Microfiche Facsimile*. Vol. 1. Binghamton, NY: Medieval & Renaissance Texts & Studies, 1994.

MacKinney, Loren. *Early Medieval Medicine*. Baltimore: The Johns Hopkins Press, 1937.

MacMahon, M. K. C. "Henry Sweet." In Helen Damico, ed. *Medieval Scholarship: Biographical Studies on the Formation of a Discipline*. Vol. 2. New York: Garland Press, 1998.

Magic and Medicine of Plants. Ninth ed. Reader's Digest Association, 1997.

Magner, Lois N. *A History of Medicine.* New York: Marcel Dekker, 1992.

Mann, John. *Murder, Magic, and Medicine.* New York: Oxford University Press, 1992.

Marcellus of Bordeaux. Max Niedermann, ed. *Marcellus Über Heilmittel.* 2 vols. Berlin: Akademie Verlag, 1968.

Maxwell, Herbert. "Odd Volumes—I." *Blackwoods Edinburgh Magazine* 163 (May 1898): 652–70.

McNeill, William H. *Plagues and Peoples.* New York: Doubleday, 1976.

Merck's Manual of the Materia Medica: A Ready Reference Pocket Book for the Practicing Physician. 1899. Reprint. New York: Merck and Co., 1999.

Miles, Frank and Graeme Cranch. *King's College School: The First 150 Years.* London: King's College School, 1979.

Minnis, A. J. *Medieval Theory of Authorship*, 2nd ed. Philadelphia: University of Pennsylvania Press, 1984.

Momma, Hal. "Old English as a Living Language: Henry Sweet and an English School of Philology." Paper presented at the annual conference of the International Society of Anglo-Saxonists, Palermo, Sicily, Italy, July 1997.

Moore, Michael. *Los Remedios de la Gente: A Compilation of Traditional New Mexican Herbal Medicines and Their Use.* Santa Fe, NM, 1977.

Morris, William. *Three Northern Love Stories and Other Tales.* Gary Aho, ed. Bristol: Thoemmes Press, 1996.

Newman, F. W. "Homeric Translation in Theory and Practice." In Matthew Arnold, *On Translating Homer: With F. W Newman's "Homeric Translation" and Arnold's "Last Words."* London: George Routledge and Sons, n.d.

Nida, Eugene A. and William D. Reyburn. *Meaning Across Cultures.* Maryknoll, NY: Orbis Books, 1981.

Ogilvy, J. D. A. *Books Known to the English, 597–1066.* Cambridge, MA: Medieval Academy of America, 1967.

Olds, Barbara. "The Anglo-Saxon Leechbook III: A Critical Edition and Translation." Ph.D. diss., University of Denver, 1984.

Papper, E. M. *Romance, Poetry, and Surgical Sleep: Literature Influences Medicine.* Westport, CT: Greenwood Press, 1995.

Payne, Joseph Frank. *The Fitz-Patrick Lectures for 1903: English Medicine in the Anglo-Saxon Times.* Oxford: Clarendon Press, 1904.

Pliny the Elder. *Natural History.* Trans. H. Rackham. 10 vols. London: Heinemann, 1938–62.

Pyles, Thomas. *The Origins and Development of the English Language.* New York: Harcourt, Brace, Jovanovich, Inc., 1970.

Richmond, Velma B. "Historical Novels to Teach Anglo-Saxonism" In Allen J. Frantzen and John D. Niles, *Anglo-Saxonism and the Construction of Social Identity.* Gainesville: University Press of Florida, 1997.

Riddle, John M. *Contraception and Abortion from the Ancient World to the Renaissance.* Cambridge, MA: Harvard University Press, 1992.

———. "Pseudo-Dioscorides' *Ex herbis femininis* and Early Medieval Medical Botany." *Journal of the History of Biology* 14 (1981), 43–81.

———. "The Textual Tradition of Dioscorides in the Latin West." In F. Edward Cranz, ed. *Catalogus Translationem et Commentanoruum* IV, 1980: 1–143.

———. "Theory and Practice in Medieval Medicine." *Viator: Medieval and Renaissance Studies* V (1974): 157–84.

Robinson, Victor. *Victory Over Pain: A History of Anesthesia.* New York: Henry Schuman, 1946.

Rose, Jeanne. *Herbs and Things: Jeanne Rose's Herbal.* New York: Workman Publishing Co., 1973.

Rubin, Stanley. *Medieval English Medicine.* New York: Barnes and Noble, 1974.

Sauer, Hans. "On the Analysis and Structure of Old and Middle English Plant Names." In *The History of English*, No. 3 (1997): 133–61.

———. "English Plant Names in the Thirteenth Century: The Trilingual Harley Vocabulary." In *Middle English Miscellany*, ed. Jacek Fisiak. Posnan: Motivex, 1996: 135–55.

———. "Towards a Linguistic Description and Classification of the Old English Plant Names." In *Words, Texts and Manuscripts: Studies in Anglo-Saxon Culture Presented to Helmut Gneuss*, ed. M. Korhammer et al. Cambridge: D.S. Brewer, 1992: 381–408.

Scragg, D. G. *Superstition and Popular Medicine in Anglo-Saxon England.* Manchester: University of Manchester, 1989.

Siegel, Rudolph E. *Galen's System of Physiology and Medicine.* Basel: S. Karger, 1968.

Sigerist, Henry E. *Studien und Texte zur frühmittelalterlichen Rezeptliteratur.* Leipzig: Verlag von J. A. Barth, 1923.

Singer, Charles. *From Magic to Science: Essays on the Scientific Twilight.* 1928. Reprint. New York: Dover Publications, 1958.

————. "The Herbal in Antiquity." *The Journal of Hellenic Studies* 47 (1927): 1–52.

Siraisi, Nancy. *Medieval and Early Renaissance Medicine.* Chicago: University of Chicago Press, 1990.

Skeat, Rev. Walter W. *A Student's Pastime: Being A Select Series of Articles Reprinted from "Notes and Queries."* Oxford: Clarendon Press, 1896.

Stanley, E. G. *The Search for Anglo-Saxon Paganism.* Cambridge: D. S. Brewer, 1975.

Stannard, Jerry. *Herbs and Herbalism in the Middle Ages and Renaissance.* London: Ashgate Variorum, 1999a.

————. *Pristina Medicamenta: Ancient and Medieval Medical Botany.* London: Ashgate Variorum, 1999b.

————. "Botanical Data and Late Mediaeval 'Rezeptliteratur.' " In Gundolf Keil. *Fachprosa-Studien: Beiträge zur mittelalterlichen Wissenschafts- und Geistesgeschichte.* Berlin: E. Schmidt, 1982.

————. "Marcellus of Bordeaux and the Beginnings of Medieval Materia Medica." *Pharmacy in History* 15, no. 2, (1973): 47–53.

Stearn, William T. *Botanical Latin.* Portand, OR: Timber Press, 1998.

Stoll, Clemens. "Arznei und Arzneiversorgung in frühmittelalterlichen Klöstern." In Gundolf Keil and Paul Schnitzer, eds. *Das Lorscher Arzneibuch und die Frühmittelalterliche Medizin: Verhandlungen des Medizinhistorischen Symposiums im September 1989 in Lorsch.* Lorsch: Verlag Laurissa, 1991.

Stoll, Ulrich. "Das Lorscher Arzneibuch: Ein Überblick über Herkunft, Inhalt und Anspruch des ältesten Arzneibuchs deutscher Provenienz." In Gundolf Keil and Paul Schnitzer, eds. *Das Lorscher Arzneibuch und die Frühmittelalterliche Medizin: Verhandlungen des Medizinhistorischen Symposiums im September 1989 in Lorsch.* Lorsch: Verlag Laurissa, 1991.

Storms, G. *Anglo-Saxon Magic.* The Hague: Martinus Nijhoff, 1974.

Stuart, Malcolm. *Encyclopedia of Herbs and Herbalism.* London: Orbis Books, 1979.

Stubbs, S. G. B. and E. W. Bligh. *Sixty Centuries of Health and Physik.* London: Sampson Low, Marsten and Co., 1931.

Sweet, Henry. Review of *Liflade of St Juliana* by Oswald Cockayne and Edmund Brock. *Academy* III, 52 (15 July 1872): 278.

————. *King Alfred's West Saxon Version of Gregory's Pastoral Care.* 1871. Reprint. London: Kegan Paul, Trench, Trübner & Co., Ltd., 1930.

————. "The History of the TH in English" (1869). In H. C. Wyld, *Collected Papers of Henry Sweet.* Oxford: Clarendon Press, 1913.

Talbot, C. H. *Medicine in Medieval England.* London: Oldbourne, 1967.

Thackeray, William M. *The History of Pendennis: His Fortunes and Misfortunes.* n.p., 1850.

Thompson, Paul. *The Work of William Morris.* 1967. Reprint. Oxford: Oxford University Press, 1993.

Thorpe, Benjamin. *Codex Exoniensis: A Collection of Anglo-Saxon Poetry, from a MS in the Library of the Dean and Chapter of Exeter.* London: n.p., 1842.

Thurston, C. B. *A Few Remarks in Defense of Dr. Bosworth and His Anglo-Saxon Dictionaries.* London: Macmillan and Co., 1864.

Tolkien, J. R. R. "*Beowulf*: The Monsters and the Critics." In *The Monsters and the Critics and Other Essays*, C. Tolkien, ed. London: George Allen & Unwin, 1983.

Tooke, John Horne. *Epea pteroenta, or the Diversions of Purley.* 1805. Richard Taylor, ed. London: Printed for Thomas Tegg, 1840.

Turner, Sharon. *The History of the Anglo-Saxons: Comprising the History of England from the Earliest Period to the Norman Conquest,* 4th ed. 3 vols. 1799–1805. Reprint. London: Longman, Hurst, Rees, Orme, and Brown, 1823.

Venn, John. *Alumni Cantabrigiensis: a biographical list of all known students, graduates and holders of office at the University of Cambridge from the earliest times to 1900.* Vol. 2. Cambridge: Cambridge University Press, 1922–27.

Venuti, Lawrence. *The Scandals of Translation: Towards an Ethics of Difference*. London: Routledge, 1998.

———. *The Translator's Invisibility: A History of Translation*. London: Routledge, 1995.

Vernon, Edward Johnston. *A Guide to the Anglo-Saxon Tongue: A Grammar after Erasmus Rask*. London: J. R. Smith, 1846.

Voigts, Linda Ehrsam. Review of *Spätantike Bilder aus der Welt des Arztes: Medizinische Bilderhandschriften der Spätantike und Ihre Mittelalterliche Überliferund* by Heide Grape-Albers. *Speculum* 57 (1982): 893–95.

———. "Anglo-Saxon Plant Remedies and the Anglo-Saxons." *Isis* 70 (1979): 250–68.

———. "The Significance of the Name Apuleius to the Herbarium Apulei." *Bulletin of the History of Medicine* 52 (1978): 214–27.

———. "A New Look at the Manuscript Containing the Old English Translation of the *Herbarium Apulei*." *Manuscripta* 20 (1976): 40–59.

———. "The Old English Herbal in Cotton MS. Vitellius C. III: Studies." Ph.D. diss., University of Missouri, 1973.

Voigts, Linda Ehrsam and Robert P. Hudson. "A drynke þat men callen dwale to make a man to slepe whyle men kerven him: A Surgical Anesthetic from Late Medieval England." In *Health, Disease and Healing in Medieval Culture*. Sheila Campbell, Bert Hall, David Klausner, eds. New York: St. Martin's Press, 1992.

Weigle, Marta and Peter White. *The Lore of New Mexico*. Albuquerque: University of New Mexico Press, 1988.

Wright, Thomas. *A Volume of Vocabularies, Illustrating the Condition and Manners of our Forefathers as well as the History of the Forms of Elementary Education and of the Languages Spoken in this Island, from the Tenth Century to the Fifteenth*. Privately Printed, 1857.

Wyld, Henry Cecil. "Henry Sweet." *Modern Language Quarterly* IV, ii (July 1901): 73–9.

Young, J. H. "Alternative Medicine in the National Institutes of Health." *Bulletin of the History of Medicine* 72 (1998): 279–98.

Index of Plant Names

The number behind the plant name refers to its chapter in the *Herbarium,* chapter 5. The Roman numerals are provided for reference to Cockayne, DeVriend, and D'Aronco and Cameron.

Name in Modern English

Agrimony, 32 (XXXII)
Alexanders, 108 (CVIII)
Alkanet, 168 (CLXVIII)
Alkanet, 42 (XLII)
Artichoke, 157 (CLVII)
Asparagus, 86 (LXXXVI)
Asphodel, 33 (XXXIII)
Asphodel, 53 (LIII)
Aster, 61 (LXI)

Barrenwort, 163 (CLXIII)
Basil, 119 (CXIX)
Basil (wild), 119 (CXIX)
Basil (sweet), 131 (CXXXI)
Betony (wood), 1 (I)
Birthwort, 20 (XX)
Bishop's weed, 164 (CLXIV)
Blackberry, 89 (LXXXIX)
Bramble, 89 (LXXXIX)
Bryony, 68 (LXVIII)
Bugloss (viper's), 161 (CLXI)

Burdock, 134 (CXXXIV)
Burdock, 37 (XXXVII)
Butcher's-broom, 59 (LIX)
Buttercup, 10 (X)

Cabbage, 130 (CXXX)
Camomile, 24 (XXIV)
Campion, 133 (CXXXIII)
Caper, 172 (CLXXII)
Caraway, 155 (CLV)
Carrot (wild), 82 (LXXXII)
Castor-oil plant, 176 (CLXXVI)
Celandine, 75 (LXXV)
Celery (wild), 120 (CXX)
Centaury, common or lesser, 36 (XXXVI)
Chervil, 106 (CVI)
Cinquefoil, 3 (III)
Cleavers, 174 (CLXXIV)
Clover (hare's-foot), 62 (LXII)
Cockspur grass, 45 (XLV)

Botanical Name

Plant Name Found in Medieval Latin Manuscripts

Old English Plant Name

Index of Medical Complaints

The numbers refer to the sections and subsections in the *Herbarium* where the complaint is mentioned. The index is fairly complete but not exhaustive.

Ache
    ear   1.4, 5.1, 19.5, 76.2, 89.1, 92.1, 132.2, 144.4, 174.2
    head   2.1, 3.4, 4.6, 54.2, 75.4, 85.1, 87.2, 90.12, 91.7, 100.2 & 8; 101.1 & 2; 119.1, 123.3, 132.1, 139.2, 143.5, 144.3, 147.2, 158.4, 169.2
    stomach   3.6, 13.1, 46.2, 59.1, 60.3, 91.3, 94.2, 106.1, 111.1, 155.1, 163.2, 184.2
    tooth   1.8, 5.3, 30.3, 76.3, 81.1, 86.2, 90.2, 97.2, 153.3, 181.3
Asthma   38.2, 42.2

Bites
    dogs   1.25, 2.21, 4.9, 37.5, 45.1, 90.15, 138.2, 177.1, 184.2
    scorpions   2.9, 64.1, 90.14, 135.4, 137.1
    snakes   1.23 & 24, 2.8, 3.7, 4.7 & 11, 6.1, 15.1, 17.1, 20.5, 25.2, 32.4, 36.1, 37.1, 63.3, 64.1, 71.1, 72.1, 89.6, 90.13 &14 & 16, 93.2, 95.1, 96.1, 98.1, 109.1, 117.5, 129.1, 135.3 & 4, 137.1, 139.3, 142.4, 143.1, 147.3, 151.1, 153.4, 155.2, 158.2, 161.1, 163.1, 173.4, 174.1
    spiders   4.8, 100.4, 139.3
    wild animals   164.1
Bladder, stones 94.8, 100.1, 136.1, 142.3, 146.3, 180.1
Blood
    (from) anus   2.5
    coughing   40.2, 134.1, 153.1

About the Author

Louis Kuykendall, Jr., D. Min., is an ordained minister in the United Church of Christ (UCC) and has served as a volunteer hospice chaplain since 2004. As a pastor in Las Vegas and Pennsylvania, Kuykendall worked with numerous youth and adults experiencing life crises. Through his service in hospice and ministry, he helps support individuals to find a place of spiritual health, hope, and acceptance. Along with his work as pastor and teacher at a local UCC parish, Kuykendall trains church and hospice volunteers to work with those facing the end of life and other spiritual and emotional challenges. He has offered presentations about hospice and spiritual care locally and nationally. Kuykendall is author of "Spiritual Health" in *Public Health Encyclopedia: Principles, People, and Programs* (ABC-CLIO). He lives with his wife Sally outside Philadelphia and enjoys tennis, reading, hiking, and traveling.

General Index

Page numbers follow entries.

Lightning Source UK Ltd.
Milton Keynes UK
UKOW06f0936060116

265882UK00016B/274/P